THE PERFECT SMILE

Tips, Tricks and Techniques to Achieve the Smile of Your Dreams

by

Dr. Joel Gould

ISBN-13: 978-1517333034

ALL DENTISTRY IS COSMETIC

About Dr. Joel Gould

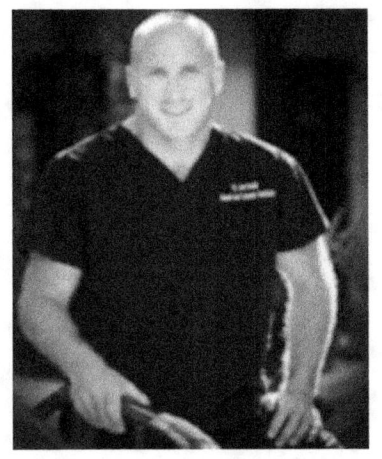

A practicing dentist for nearly 25 years, Dr. Joel Gould has provided his outstanding services in the Southern California area since 2001. His general and cosmetic dental team treats patients of all ages and offers a broad range of comprehensive oral medical care. Dr. Gould owned and operated several dental practices in Vancouver, Canada, for over a decade before relocating to the United States.

In addition to his primary dental work, Dr. Gould has trained with several top Beverly Hills plastic surgeons in the art, science, and application of Botox˚ and Juvéderm˚ facial fillers. This expertise enables him to provide his patients with a one-stop solution for beautiful dentofacial esthetic treatments to achieve his signature Perfect Smile Makeover. He has also collaborated with Dmitriy's Dental Studios to create the "Supermodel Veneer," which he utilizes in both his Instant Smile Makeovers and Instant Pageant Makeovers.

Dr. Gould recently launched his new practice and concept called Modern American Dentistry˚, which is a straightforward and innovative approach to practice that he and his team routinely employ to create a consistently comfortable and effective dental experience for his patients. The locations of Modern American Dentistry include the flagship Manhattan Beach, California, office and those in Northridge and Santa Monica. Dr. Gould's practices have treated over a quarter-million patients in both Canada and the United States. He has placed thousands of cosmetic dental restorations and has developed new critical cosmetic dental products. He also writes a regular column on cosmetic dentistry for Pageantry Magazine, which is distributed in 52 countries around the world.

Dedication

This book is dedicated to my parents. I am saddened that they are not here to see this book become a reality.

With their love, support, and dedication, I was able to attain a great education, focus clearly on my career, and create my dream dental company.

Table of Contents

Introduction

Most dentists graduate from dental school and, soon after, find a good associateship in a suitable location to practice. They usually remain there until a principal dentist retires, and subsequently step in to take over the care of the practice's patients. Unlike those dentists, I have never taken the traditional route in my career. All of the unusual twists and turns that my dental career has taken, and every failed opportunity that seemed like a reasonable choice at the time, ultimately became the catalyst for the "aha" moment I had a few years ago. At that time, I was focused on the daily struggle of running multiple dental practices and training associate dentists at my offices. One of my associate dentists, Dr. Gabe Adorjan, called me to discuss a case that was a bit complex, which is something all of my associates are encouraged to do. After we collaborated, I lamented over an online review that was less than positive.

Dr. Gabe told me in no uncertain terms that I was way out of line, focusing on the few negative complaints we receive from time to time. These complaints arise mostly because of a lack of communication. Most of what I believe in, do, and instruct my associate dentists to do, is preventive in nature. Placing a filling before decay reaches a nerve and causes pain, replacing a small failing filling before a tooth fractures and requires a more expensive crown, or placing a crown on a large failing filling before it fractures, requiring a much more expensive implant, are examples of this philosophy. Because teeth won't hurt during the early stages of dental disease (gum disease and cavities), patients can become upset with us when a procedure is recommended *before* pain is felt, and due to the nature of restorative dentistry, common complications can be a bit uncomfortable for a short time.

Dr. Gabe asked me, "Do you know how many people you have helped? Do you understand how much money, time, and pain you have saved all of your patients?"

Those comments truly helped me to see the big picture that I had lost sight of in the course of the daily grind. The truth is that dentistry is often a thankless career. Most people genuinely hate to go to the dentist. Over and over again, I have heard so many shocking stories and listened to so many patients recount their bad dental experiences. On that fateful day on the telephone, however, a trusted friend and colleague helped me to remember what I really love about my profession: changing someone's perception of dentistry.

I have taken all of the best dental procedures and protocols from my entire career, broken them down, and reassembled them to their best incarnation. I have created a unique contemporary program that all of my teams in each of my practices follow. This model of practice values long-term relationships over profit, with my belief that honesty is the only way to practice. Ultimately, the uniquely intimate nature of dentistry requires that patients place their trust in us. It's really a collaboration between dentist and patient. I believe it is our duty to educate our patients through the use of digital X-rays, clear intra-oral photographs, effective discussions, and easy-to-understand digital resources and content on our website www.modernamericandentistry.com so that treatment is obvious to all.

My concept is
Modern American Dentistry® (MAD).

Why MAD? I have worked at many dental offices over the decades and I have seen countless patients who'd stayed for many years with one dentist who had essentially had failed them. Simply stated, I was MAD at my profession. What I have seen makes me mad because dentistry has changed so dramatically and has evolved in an amazing way. The problem is that the evolution I have worked so hard to see and participate in has left many dentists behind as their careers came closer to an end. The most common and damaging problem I see and have seen is the lack of a common-sense, organized, consistent system, and protocols that help dentists to run an efficient, respectful dental practice in which all patients receive appropriate, and timely treatment. Dentists don't always agree what those systems, protocols, and treatment recommendations are, and that is OK. Dentistry is too personal, and people are too different to have a one-size-fits-all solution, or a "*CAN* please all of the people all of the time*"* result.

My goal with Modern American Dentistry is to supply and teach a simple, organized, efficient set of rules, regulations, procedures, and protocols, to try to simplify the delivery of great oral health.

A new way isn't necessarily always better. Some tried-and-true procedures need to remain the same and be routinely utilized. My interest is really more about how patients are being treated. Often, dentists focus on small procedures, rather than on the big picture. I have seen dentists fail to educate their patients and enlist their understanding of how their mouth needs to be maintained. From not taking appropriate X-rays to failing to maintain patient records to not recommending preventive treatment coordinated with dental-insurance benefits, I have seen it all. As dental-health professionals, we are charged with the responsibility to do right for our patients. We are altering a human being's body. With that comes an unwavering respect for the patient and an ongoing commitment to their personal dental health—starting on day one. I have always, and will always, train all of my dentists to respect all people.

Who Am I?

Over the past 25 years, I have become adept in general and cosmetic dentistry. In addition to my legal status as a DDS, my core background includes continuing-education classes, hands-on training, medical lectures, and a lifetime of experience in the field of dentistry. My professional experience includes, but is not limited to, the following general and cosmetic dental practices, as well as related activities:

- Public-health dentistry
- Mobile dental treatment to underserved areas
- Pediatric dental practice
- Geriatric dental practice
- Hospital dentistry, including pediatric and adult unconscious sedation
- Practice acquisition, recreation, and transformation
- Start-up and founding of new practices
- Supervision of new-practice construction
- Relocation of existing practices
- Successful sale of transformed practices
- Transition of retired dentists and assimilation of new dental staff
- Marketing
- Employment
- Mentoring
- Renovation
- Branding
- Creation of systems, protocols, and unique time-saving procedures
- Innovation of dentofacial and related antiaging esthetic techniques
- Advanced, multidisciplinary full-mouth reconstruc-

tion
- Public speaking
- Writing articles to educate the public about dentistry
- Involvement in charities

The many facets of my career in dentistry are my life's work. The creation of Modern American Dentistry reflects my own experiences, both as a dentist and a patient, as well as those of friends and family, and my colleagues' past successes and failures. I have experienced a diverse and large number of professional dental-practice scenarios over the years. As such, I wanted to create the dental practice and philosophy of my dreams to show the world that today the modern practice of dentistry is something more, something better, and something much easier to embrace.

My goal is to enable patients to see and understand dentistry as I do. I intend to achieve the following:

- Change patients' perceptions of pain or discomfort that they have experienced in the past and allow them to evolve from a position of fear and dread to one of understanding and acceptance.
- Help patients trust their dentist and their dental office, as well as lift fears surrounding the intimate and anxiety-provoking aspect of oral health.
- Provide a high practice standard, whereby patients expect a uniform, comfortable, and consistent experience, regardless of the individual provider or dental-office location. I especially seek to impart the knowledge that we can provide deep and thorough anesthesia so patients will experience no pain during their procedure.
- Provide consistent and predictable outcomes for all procedures and dental visits, as well as supply proper

and realistic postoperative instruction and support for complications very common to many dental procedures.

- Raise the "dental IQ" of our patients and attract patients who value their health and trust our guidance through understandable patient-education modalities. These include easy-to-comprehend preoperative and postoperative information, photography and X-rays that utilize dynamic technology, our website and app, and the ability of our team members to easily explain our work and their experience.

- Simplify and standardize the often-confusing financial aspect of dental insurance and estimates, as well as facilitate the acceptance of treatment. We will seek to help patients most effectively utilize their insurance benefits and monies to be spent on oral health.

- Stay current and utilize appropriate dental technology where it is necessary and beneficial, rather than follow fads or trends created by dental-industry advertising.

- Simplify and make convenient all aspects of patients' home care and dental regimens, including the provision of written and digital information, as well as useful dental products that we research, recommend, and provide for sale at our offices.

- And, most of all, provide respectful, honest, and thorough dental care, as well as the management of patients' oral health over the years.

My vision of what dentistry is and should be today is Modern American Dentistry.

Joel Gould

THE PERFECT SMILE

All Dentistry Is Cosmetic

Everyone has developed an individual idea of what his or her perfect smile would look like. There is no one-size-fits-all answer. A person's smile is so directly integrated into his or her personality and how he or she perceives his or her overall image that it is difficult to lay out a formula for perfection. Looking in the mirror daily, most people can find something that is not exactly perfect about their smile, which is OK because variation is great! What I routinely see in my dental practice is a mixture of people who are relatively happy with their smile, but who would like to modify one aspect of it, such as: "I wish I had whiter teeth" or "I have some crowding in my lower front teeth and I am interested in hearing about what can be done to correct it."

I do see many patients who arrive at my office after having performed some online research. They all say the same thing: "I hate my smile and I always cover my mouth when I speak or laugh." These are my favorite patients, as they provide me with an opportunity to transform their smiles—and their lives! Often, their resultant unhappiness has affected their self-esteem. This category of patient needs more than a quick fix; they need a dentist to help walk them down the road to the smile that they have always wanted but are unsure of even how to open a dialogue with their dentist. These patients are often the victims of what I call "smile dissonance." The teeth and smile they have are no longer an appropriate fit for who they have become inside and as a person. These are individuals who have achieved a high level of success and confidence in their lives, yet retain the mismatched smile of their youth—a smile that doesn't portray who they have become. This is usually characterized by heavily restored and discolored teeth, missing teeth, or poorly arranged teeth. Recognizing these patients isn't always easy, as they have "managed" over the years, but have most likely been unhappy with their smile since they can remember.

There is no list or combination of dental treatments that will result in a perfect smile every time. In the following pages, you will find a summary of dental procedures and explanations that should help you become better informed about dentistry as you learn that, effectively, *all dentistry is cosmetic.*

I hope that this book will inspire you, the reader and dental patient, to feel empowered and comfortable about having a constructive dialogue with your own dentist. My goal is to inform and motivate you enough to help you to define what treatment is needed in order to help you decide exactly what *your* perfect smile looks like.

Smile Assessment

This is the most important step in changing your smile. I wrote this book to make it easier for you, the patient, to be able to tell your dentist what you don't like about your smile. Tear out of magazines any pages that portray teeth, lips, and smiles that you like! I have even seen patients who told me they wanted to look like superstar Angelina Jolie, which is great, as this can, at least, give a dentist an idea about your expectations.

Maybe you don't need a full dental makeover. Maybe you'd just like whiter teeth or less crowding. After reading this, I hope that you will be able to tell your dentist exactly what it is about your smile that you want to change.

The first thing that should be done is a "smile assessment." It can be really informal and simple, and should include a hand mirror, so that you can point out any areas in your mouth with which you are not happy. Your dentist should be able to guide you through the process and ask some questions to get a better idea of what you want to change. Understanding the elements of the perfect smile is a critical step in creating the smile of your dreams.

The Elements of a Smile

The three key components that come together to create the smile of your dreams are the teeth, lips, and lower face. A balanced combination of these elements works to achieve a perfect smile.

- ## Face and Lips

Before I get to the starring role of this book and the area of expertise that dentists focus upon—the teeth—it is important to discuss the face and lips. The lips frame the mouth and cannot be left out of any cosmetic dentistry discussion. I will limit the content here and simply say that when it comes to lip support, the positioning of the teeth is critical, and they ultimately contribute to how the lips and face will rest against these hard structures.

The lip line, or bottom of the upper lip, is critical when it comes to how much tooth structure is revealed. The lip line is a moving target; we see much more of the lower teeth as people age. A youthful smile almost always shows two millimeters of the upper front teeth extending past the upper lip at rest, or during speech. We want to see much more of the teeth when we smile. As we age, what we end up with isn't always attractive. My concept of antiaging dentistry uses all dental-treatment modalities to keep an appropriately youthful smile. The use of dermal fillers, such as Juvéderm˚, is where dentistry needs to focus. Multiple techniques can be used to maintain a natural smile at any age. In my practice, I only use techniques and materials that are completely reversible, because as we age, our bodies change. As a result, I must adapt to those changes with different and more appropriate techniques. What looks great in someone's 20s may appear inappropriate in his or her 50s.

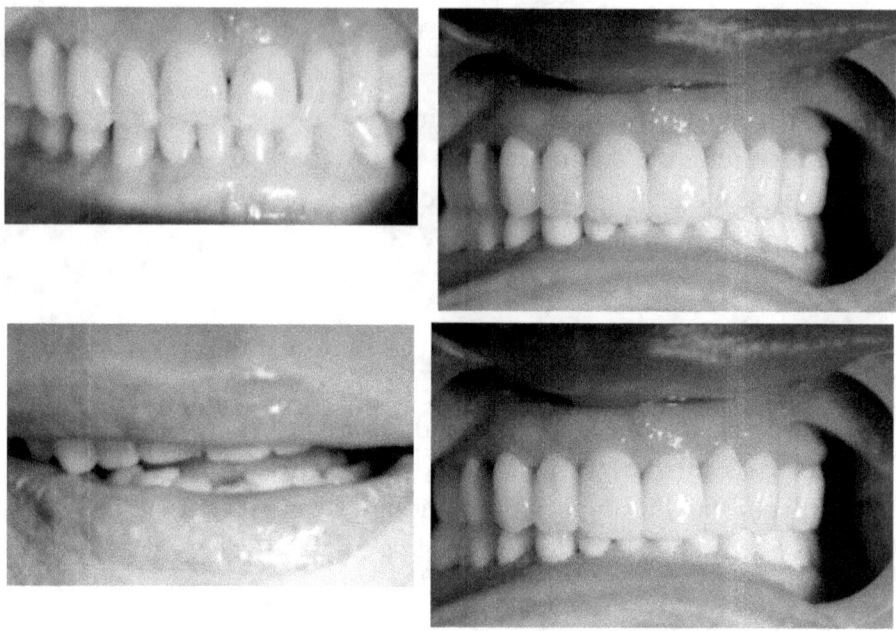

Before and After, Full-Mouth Reconstruction

To create the perfect smile, dentists sometimes use materials, such as dermal fillers like Juvéderm˚, to augment the lips and lower face. Juvéderm˚, in men and women, plumps lips, reduces lines, and reshapes the tissues around the mouth to restore volume and a youthful appearance. Occasionally, Botox˚ is used in very limited applications to partially paralyze facial muscles; it is primarily reserved for the upper face, eyes, and forehead.

Not all dentists are trained in the use of dermal fillers, and it's best to seek help from more than one provider should you feel you would benefit from these safe and fantastic products.

Antiaging dentistry is common-sense preventive dentistry. When prevention isn't an option, we can turn back the clock by utilizing all of the treatment options I will discuss in this book.

Teeth Simplified

We assess teeth within three very specific categories: Arrangement, Color and Translucency, and Shape.

• Arrangement

In a perfect world, all teeth are well aligned and are arranged in a balanced, curved arch, blending harmoniously with the other structures of the jaw, such as the gums and bone that support the teeth. Plainly put, ideally arranged teeth are very attractive. Aligned teeth wear better and are easier to clean, resulting in better periodontal health. Misaligned teeth often wear very unevenly, causing unusual and destructive wear on certain teeth. When all of the teeth are in an ideal setup, or alignment, chewing will not destroy any tooth structure prematurely, and the teeth will ultimately last longer and remain in better shape. When teeth are well aligned, it's easier to remove plaque and tarter, which always results in better periodontal health.

Teeth become misaligned for many reasons, starting from as early as birth due to prolonged thumb sucking or even pacifier use. Genetics also play a huge role in how the teeth emerge and move into place. The whole process of children losing their baby teeth and gaining their adult teeth that move into place is a hugely complex set of circumstances and functions. In the dental world, we simplify the complexity of final adult-tooth positioning by calling it "multifactorial." (That means it's really complicated and highly variable.) Children's growth, nutrition, genetics, and habits can create an arrangement that often does not look great. Words like "overbite" and "bucktoothed" are often used as insults in school, and developing personalities can be harshly affected or scarred for life.

The simplest and often most conservative way to correct misaligned teeth falls into the category known as "orthodontics." When we want teeth to be placed somewhere different than where they currently exist, we exert a force on teeth in the direction that we want them to move. Pressure exerted against bone will cause a cellular function called "bone reabsorption" (cells called "osteoclasts" erode bone, allowing a tooth to move forward). Behind the tooth, a different cellular function called "bone apposition" occurs, (different cells called "osteoblasts" create new bone to fill in behind the tooth) and new bone will occupy the space where the tooth used to be. This allows us to slowly move teeth through bone to almost any location. As we move teeth, the surrounding gum tissue will slowly remodel itself and move with the tooth to the new position.

• Orthodontics

Certified orthodontists are best suited to treating children as they grow and develop into adults. Complex tooth growth patterns can be difficult to manage and unless a general dentist has substantial orthodontic training and experience beyond dental school, I feel it is best left to a highly trained specialist. General dentists do very well in treating simple cases of tooth crowding, cosmetic tooth correction, and other minor problems. All orthodontic procedures include both fixed and removable devices to control tooth movement.

Although there are still some cases that require fixed brackets (old-school braces), a very large number of orthodontic cases can be successfully treated by using clear aligners, such as ClearCorrect˙ and Invisalign˙. Clear aligners have so many advantages over fixed brackets that, in my opinion, they have become the modern evolution of what we used to call braces. My desire to modernize dentistry fits perfectly with this more recent technological development.

• Fixed Brackets

Metal or white ceramic brackets are cemented to teeth and hold wires and elastic bands to move teeth into the ideal position.

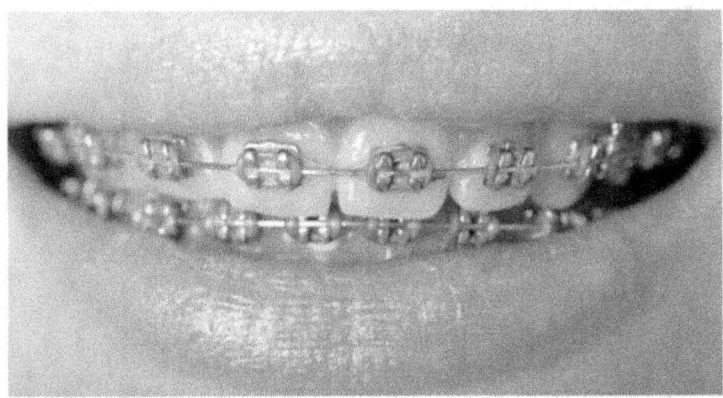

• Clear Aligners

Patients wear clear, plastic, custom-fit trays on their teeth. The dentist or orthodontist uses a unique computer application to generate a start-to-finish treatment plan, and a dental laboratory fabricates the clear aligners. They are to be worn for at least 22 hours a day, and are changed out at home about every two weeks. Often a mid-treatment revision is required before the treatment is complete.

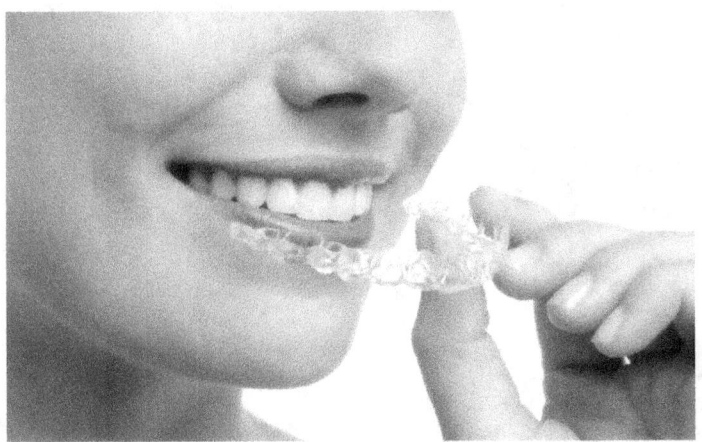

Modern technology has given rise to a device that, when used properly, will reduce ANY orthodontic treatment by almost half; it's called the Accelodent. This device vibrates at a certain frequency stimulating increased blood flow. The result? All cellular functions involved in moving teeth are amplified; helping us achieve the final-result you're looking for faster than ever.

Both types of orthodontics require a "retention phase" to solidify the new position of the teeth, achieved by wearing retainers initially at all times and then just at night. Retainers are critical, as almost all orthodontic work dentists perform in general practice is to correct a previously treated case that has relapsed.

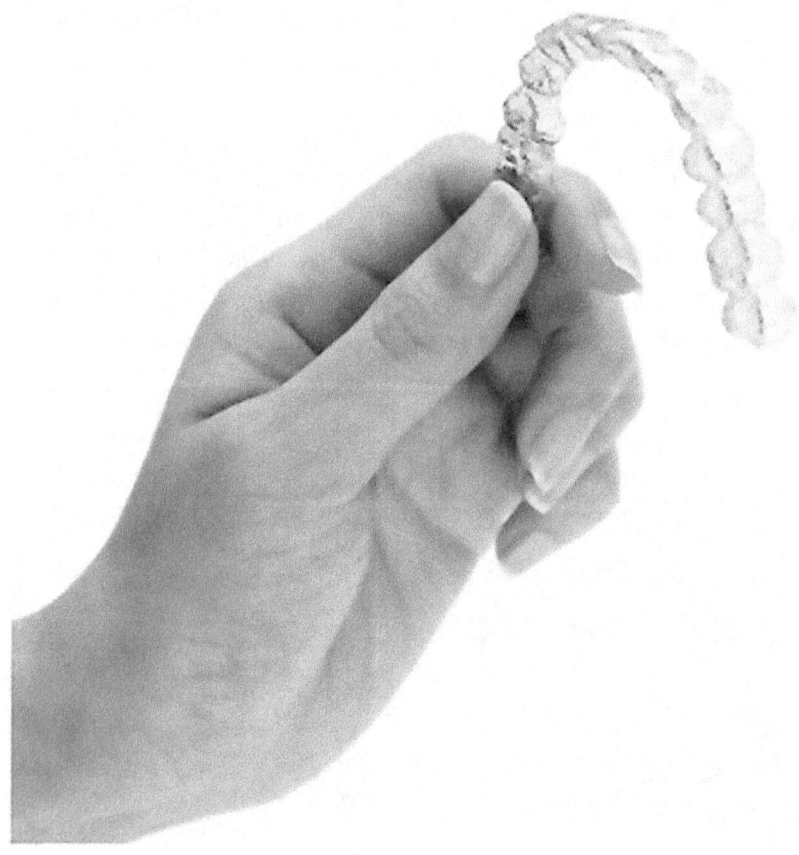

The clear aligner revolution has transformed modern cosmetic dentistry, as adults at almost any age are much more receptive to "orthodontics" as long as they do not need to wear visible metal brackets.

The most fantastic part of   clear aligners is their ability to allow patients to keep their teeth clean without any special or difficult regimen, such as using a "floss threader" to get between teeth. There are no periods of adjustment where the metal brackets cut the lips until scar tissue forms. Aligners are comfortable from day one.

• Other Ways to Correct Tooth Arrangement

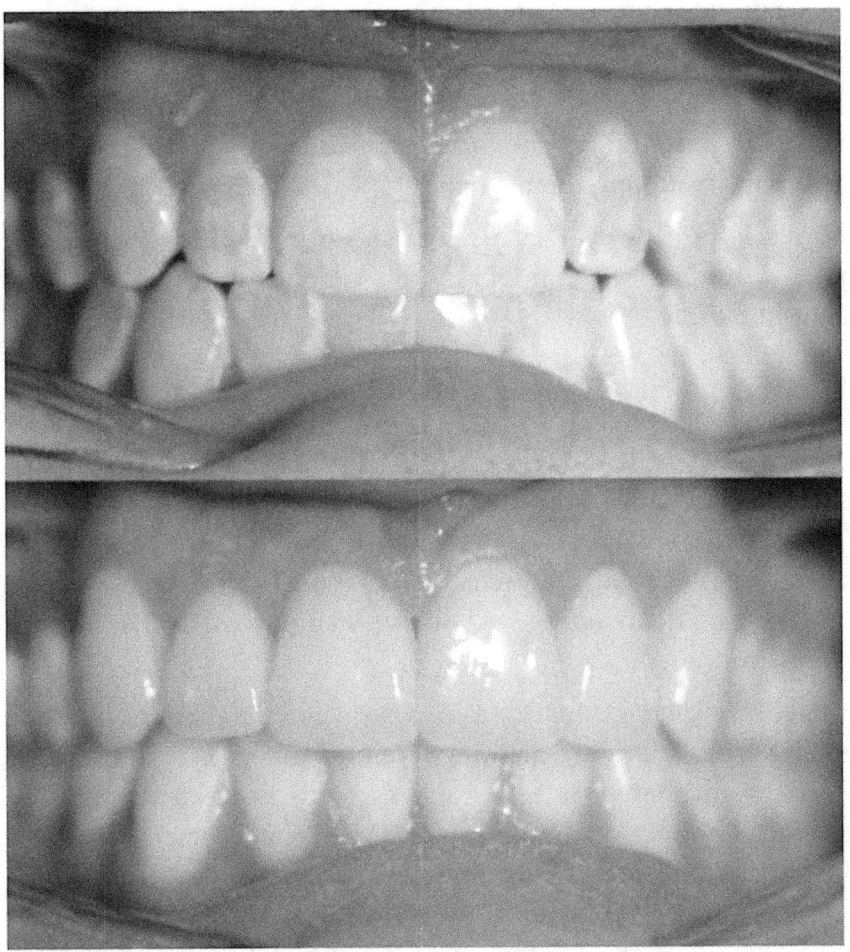

When a patient has small teeth and a large jaw or a small jaw and large teeth, known as "tooth-arch-size discrepancy," it may be physically impossible to achieve good alignment, no matter how skilled a dentist orthodontist is. In these cases, as well as in situations where orthodontics are not possible or where there are missing or damaged teeth that require restoration, we need to consider what modern dentistry has to offer by way of esthetic and restorative treatments. Also, if the tooth shape, size, and color are not ideal, we should consider enhancing a patient's smile with a cosmetic restoration. Directly bonded composite filling material, known as "bonding," can alter the shape, size, and color of teeth. We can also consider the use of crowns, veneers, and implants to change the arrangement of the teeth to a more ideal appearance.

We have established tooth arrangement as critical to a beautiful smile, and orthodontics can greatly transform a patient's smile by simply moving teeth into their proper

locations. However, if having a beautiful smile was as easy as that, I would be out of a job and everyone would feel great about his or her smile.

• Color

Kids don't lie. If you want to know if your teeth are too dark or too yellow, just ask a five-year-old. Their filter isn't yet ready to spare your feelings, and it's not a bad thing. It has inspired thousands of my own patients to ask about what we can do to whiten their teeth. Of course, you can also ask an adult loved one, as well as your dentist, about the color of your teeth.

Genetics play a huge role in what a person's teeth will end up looking like. There are also many environmental factors that can affect the ultimate shade or color of teeth, such as during development. The teeth of many people who used certain antibiotics, like tetracycline, are often stained because of the medication. Many teenaged or adult patients these days have discoloration from too much fluoride during a tooth's formation, called fluorosis. Minor fluorosis cases can be treated with microabrasion, which consists of polishing superficial stains with abrasives.

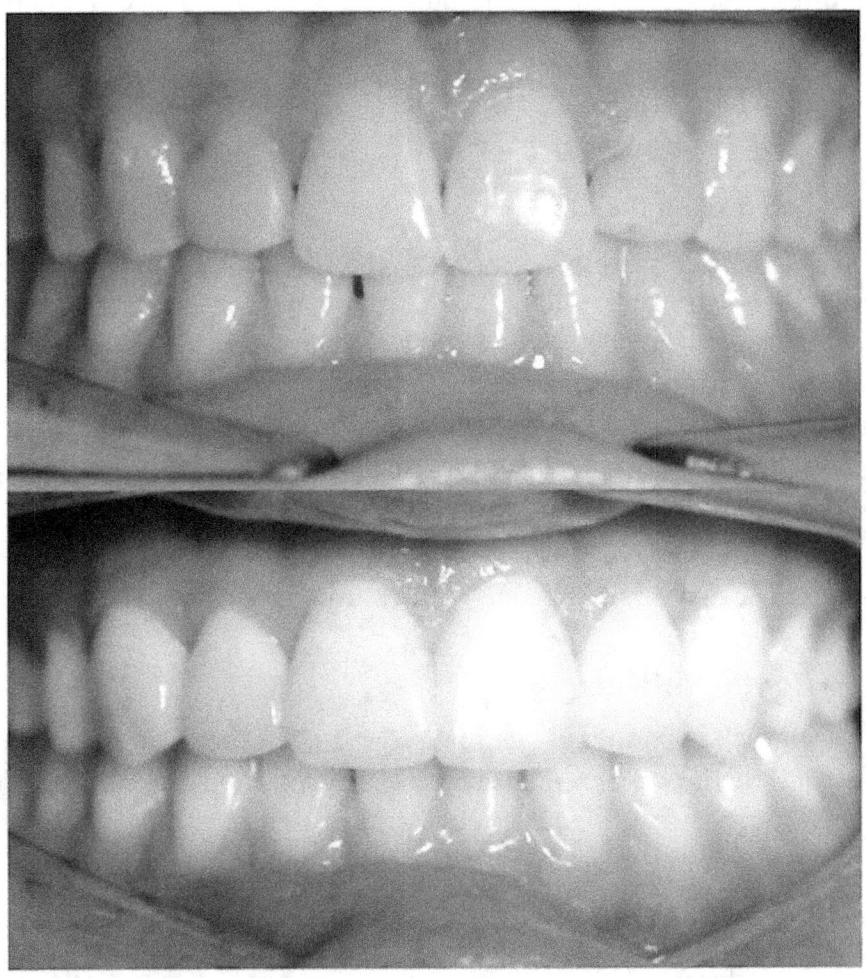

Daily environmental factors also act to darken and stain the enamel of our teeth, such as drinking red wine, eating dark berries, and, of course, drinking coffee. This section of the book isn't about breaking down hue, value, and chroma. That's for dentists and artists to learn and know. But what is the solution to discolored teeth?

• Daily Home Care

Electric toothbrushes and devices such as flossers have helped to modernize how we clean our teeth, making it easier than ever to keep teeth clean and healthy. The Philips Sonicare™ is an electric tooth-brush that we recommend to our patients, since the patented vibration action goes a long way to remove stains and keep teeth as white as possible.

• Professional Care

Yes, cleanings every six months are critical for dental health, as even the best brushers and flossers need to have every surface of every tooth cleaned at and below the gum line by a dental hygienist or dentist. This is performed to remove calcium deposits, which harbor harmful bacteria. We actually recommend upward of three to four cleanings per year, although dental insurance often only pays for two per year. It is up to the individual patient to decide what is right for him or her.

At the end of your cleaning appointment, a "polish" with a light pumice is usually performed to remove any surface stain.

• Tooth Whitening

All of the products listed below will work well when they are used according to the manufacturer's recommendations. Due to the variations of patient genetics and environmental factors, results will vary from individual to individual. I have read claims by companies about their products' ability to make teeth 5-to-10 shades whiter. I feel that this is very subjective, and there are several different shade guides that can be used to measure tooth color and tone results.

Studies have also shown over the years that almost all tooth bleaching or whitening procedures work. They contain some proprietary mixture of ingredients, along with the active ingredients of either hydrogen peroxide or carbamide peroxide.

Whitening products come in a huge variety of applications and dosages. Below, you will find a simplified list of what's available and the products we most frequently use or recommend at any of my Modern American Dentistry locations.

• **Crest° Whitestrips**—These bleaching strips are shockingly effective, easy to use, and very convenient.

Advantage: Low cost and ease of use

Disadvantage: Sensitivity, which can be severe, and the need for multiple applications

• **Opalescence° Go**—This teeth-whitening system is comprised of easy, one-size-fits-all, take-home bleach trays that effectively deliver a whitening formula to the enamel of the teeth.

Advantage: Cost, easy to use, disposable, and gentle for those with tooth sensitivity

Disadvantage: Requires repeat applications

• **Take-Home Custom Teeth Trays**—These custom-fitted trays are made with a small reservoir for patients to apply gel bleach. Patients fit them in their mouths for between 30 minutes and one hour.

Disadvantage: Higher cost and repeat applications

• In-Office Whitening

Many dental product and material companies market their systems for "in-office" or "one-hour, take-home" whitening use. They all typically work. I have not seen any specific system that is truly superior. It is important to keep in mind that there is a huge competitive marketing component to these products. After all, who can blame the companies that produce them? They want to sell their products. That said, it is comforting to know that these companies have spent time, attention, and money to ensure that their products and procedures are safe and effective.

I have used all of these teeth-whitening systems at some point in my career. We currently offer both Philips Zoom and Opalescence° at my Modern American Dentistry locations. On a side note, I prefer not to use the BriteSmile° system due to their contractual obligations, but it works as well as any of the major brands on the market today.

Some of these teeth-whitening systems use a bright light that follows the application of a viscus gel to teeth. Studies have shown that these systems are not necessarily more effective when the light is used, while other studies claim that the heat emitted from the light is very traumatic to tooth nerves. I prefer not to use it unless a patient makes a specific request, as my experience has shown that it can cause more tooth sensitivity.

Disadvantages of this type of whitening are usually minor and very temporary. They include burns on the gums, on which we suggest applying vitamin E oil to help the tissue heal. Severe temperature sensitivity is common, as well as very powerful electric-shock sensations, both of which are usually limited to the day of the procedure, and are easily relieved by a combination of Tylenol® and ibuprofen.

Over-bleaching will result in tooth enamel becoming too translucent and taking on a grey shade that is not appealing. I see this most often in patients who use take-home products too frequently.

• Maintenance of Tooth Shade

Avoiding dark, staining foods, and using a Philips Sonicare® toothbrush can help keep your teeth looking lighter/whiter.

• Translucency

Along with color, there is another component of tooth appearance, called "translucency," which enables light to pass through an object. Natural teeth are very translucent in that they transmit a lot of light. Teeth that are more opaque, on the other hand, can look fake. It's a critical part of cosmetic dentistry to make sure that

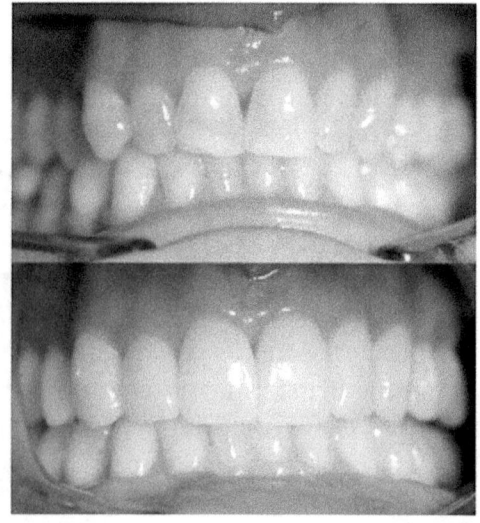

teeth appear lifelike when a patient smiles! Translucency is also essential to achieve when performing restorations such as porcelain veneers and crowns. While translucency varies from person to person, all teeth need to exhibit some degree of light transmission.

It's the job of the dentist and technician to either match your own translucency—so a restoration blends well—or to create a natural-looking level and style of translucency for multiple restorations. (This is when photographs of teeth a patient loves or wants to recreate would be beneficial.)

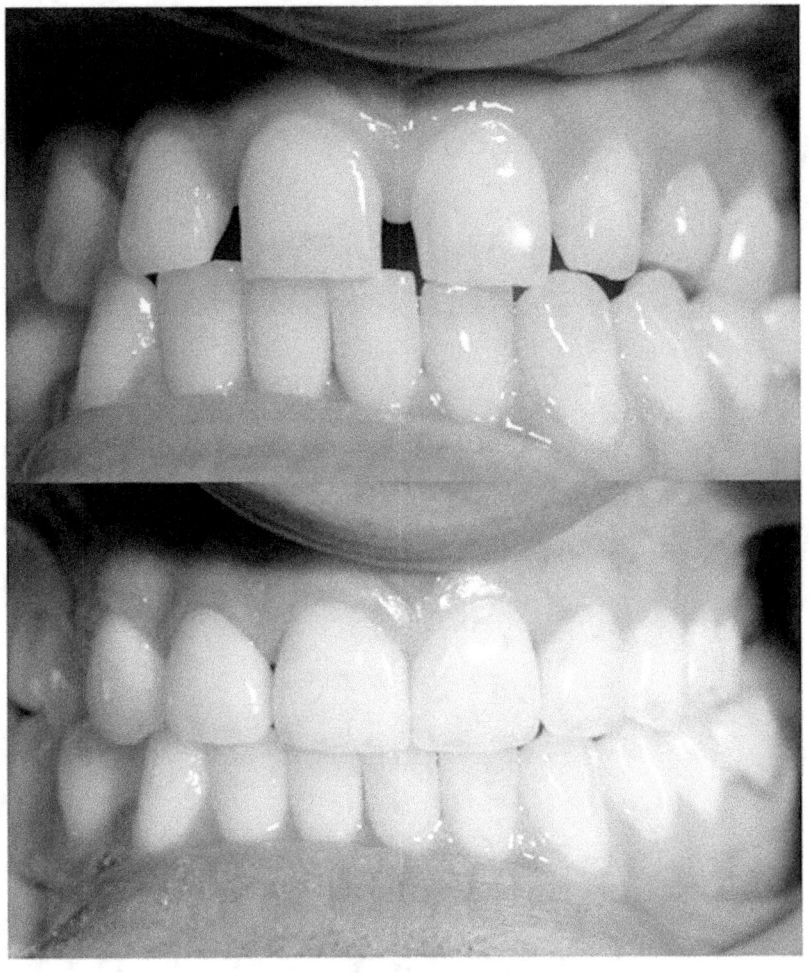

Six Porcelain Crowns

Shape

"Shape" is a simple word for a complex topic. People have uniquely-shaped teeth due to a combination of factors, such as genetics, wear, and restorations. This area is where all of the complex restorative dental-treatment modalities come into play. I wanted to simplify this topic, but it is anything but simple! Below, I will lay out the various cosmetic and functional ways that dentists restore smiles. I discussed "antiaging dentistry," and a large component of that topic falls into maintaining, or re-establishing, a patient's proper lip support. Dental restorative treatments can restore a person's face and lip support to create the smile of anyone's dreams by replacing or restoring lost teeth or tooth structure.

Cosmetic Restorations

When orthodontics and whitening your own natural teeth aren't an option, dentists will utilize restorations such as crowns, veneers, or direct composite filling material to modify the appearance of a tooth. By using these restorations, we can change the size, shape, color and arrangement of a tooth. We can redistribute the spaces between teeth to make them more Ideal. For example, if a patient has spaces between their teeth, or diastema, like pop singer Madonna, veneers or crowns can be made wider to narrow those gaps.

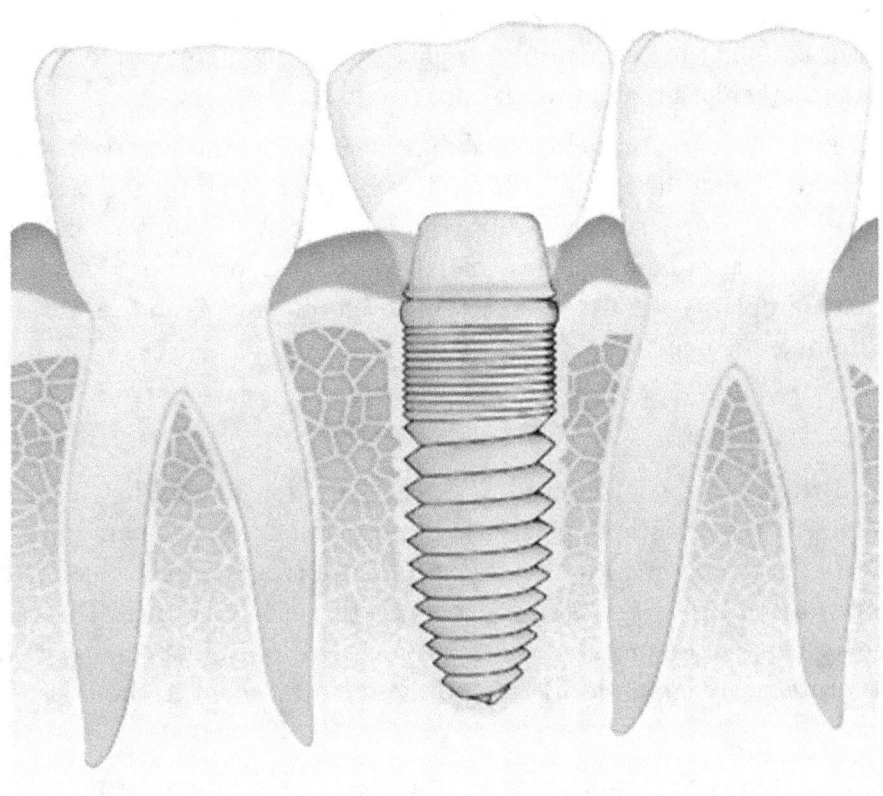

• Implants

Dentists use dental implants to replace missing teeth. General dentists place implants, but often refer to a periodontist or an oral surgeon if the placement is complicated. The first stage is to place a titanium implant that is shaped like a root into the bone of the jaw. It can take up to six months for the implant to "integrate" into bone.

Often, due to previous gum disease and bone loss, a bone graft may be required before there is sufficient room for an implant to stay in the jaw for the long term. This is done fairly painlessly and easily, and can provide a great foundation for a whole new tooth.

A metal or white zirconia connector called an abutment is placed into the implant and the part of the abutment that sticks up past the gums is fitted for a crown. A well-placed dental implant can look and feel exactly like a regular tooth once completed.

Implants can also help to stabilize a partial denture, or even a full denture, so that the fit can withstand heavy chewing. Implants can also anchor or secure partial or full dentures to provide comfort and security, and eliminate unsightly metal clasps used to anchor a denture. Dental implants can also be mixed in with both crowns and veneers to eliminate the need for a bridge.

• Bridges

Bridges can also be used to replace missing teeth. They are cemented permanently in place and can drastically affect a person's appearance by creating ideal teeth alignment. Bridges require that teeth on either side of the missing tooth, or teeth, receive a crown. This can be destructive to a totally healthy unrestored tooth, but can be great to protect any large old fillings on the teeth adjacent to the missing tooth.

A bridge consists of at least three teeth, where the missing tooth gets replaced with a false tooth attached to full crowns on either side of the space (called a "pontic"). Once cemented, the bridge is pretty much indistinguishable from other completely natural teeth, and cannot be easily removed. Bridges can restore multiple missing teeth, but implants are being used much more frequently in today's modern dental world.

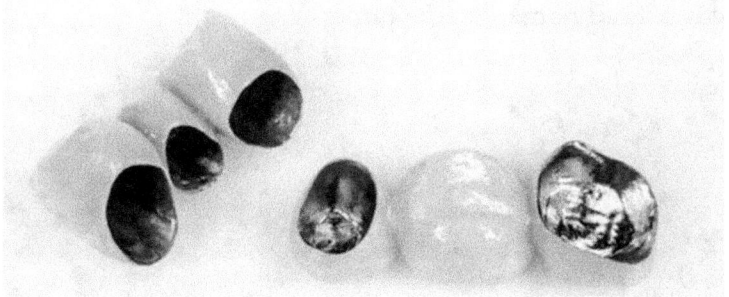

• Dentures

When multiple teeth are missing, dentists can fabricate partial or complete removable dentures that can attach to adjacent teeth or to dental implants placed in strategic locations in the jaw bone.

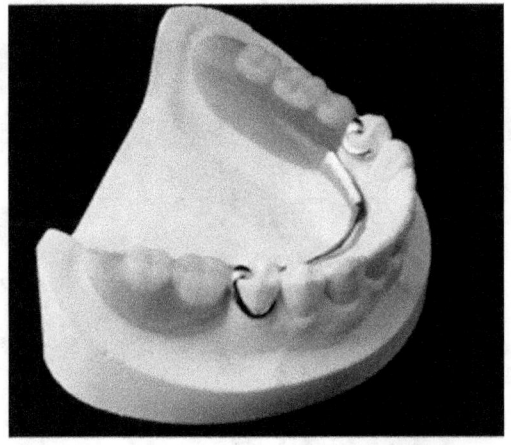

Your dentist is best suited to review with you these options for tooth replacement. While removable devices will not be discussed here, it is another topic I hope to cover in future publications.

• Bonding

Bonding is what dentists refer to when they use composite resin, the white filling material that is used to replace silver amalgams in most modern offices. This same filling material can be placed on front teeth in moderate amounts, or for temporary results, until a more permanent material, like porcelain can be used to replace it. A great example of its use is for anyone under the age of 21. Since young adults are still growing, and the gums are rapidly changing, it is often better to use bonding for cosmetic results. It is temporary and can be fully removed without damaging the underlying teeth.

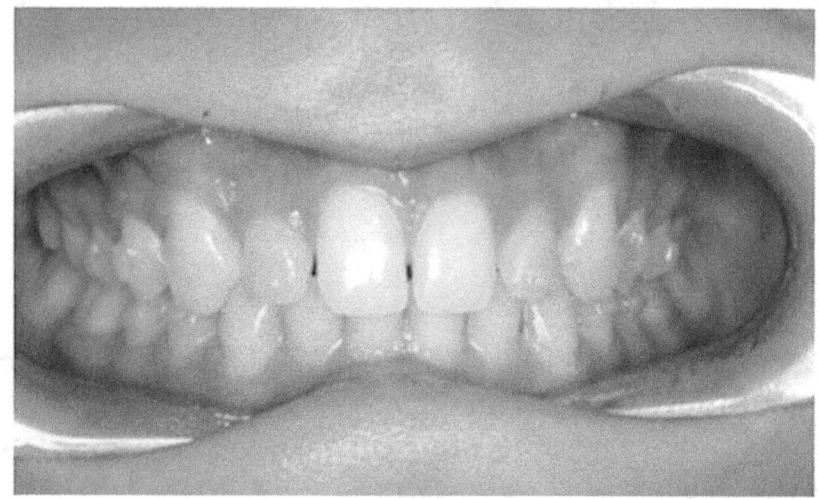

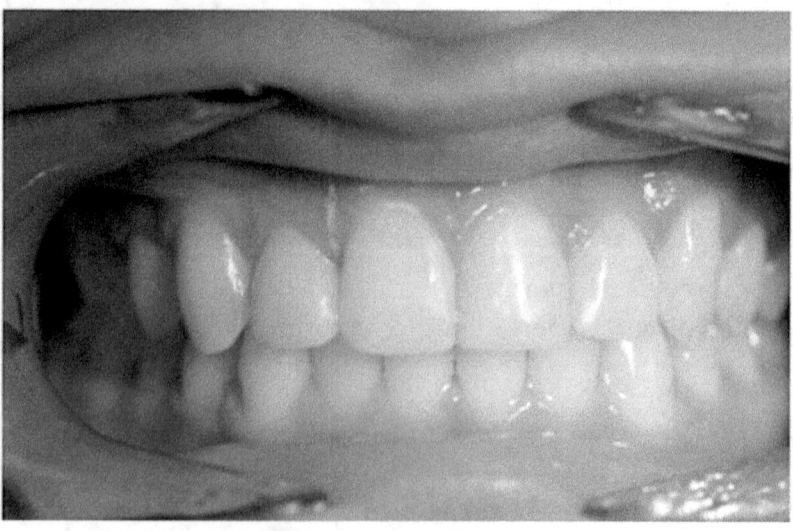

Before and After Cosmetic Bonding on a 16-Year-Old

• Crowns and Veneers

Porcelain veneers and crowns are restorations that can completely transform a tooth by altering its color, shape, and orientation. Esthetic porcelain restorations can be made to look like virtually anything.

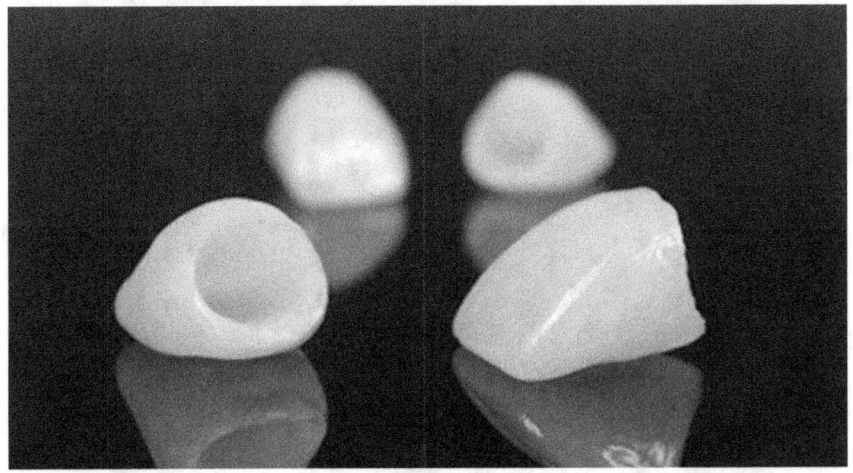

All-Ceramic Crowns

The difference between crowns and veneers is that a crown protects the entire tooth being treated, and a veneer is a restoration that covers primarily the front part of the tooth.

A dentist will choose a crown or a veneer based on certain results that are desired. The basic difference for their use is how much protection a tooth needs. Crowns are used as a "restorative" technique to reinforce or fortify a tooth that has been broken down by trauma or a tooth that has been filled many times and no longer has enough tooth structure to be structurally sound. Even though the big difference between crowns and veneers is how they are attached to the tooth (the veneer is bonded and the crown is cemented), crowns can also be bonded with adhesive cements. This is often done to improve the retention of a crown, making it harder to remove a crown that has been bonded. This technique can be used on small or short teeth to enhance the long-term retention of a crown.

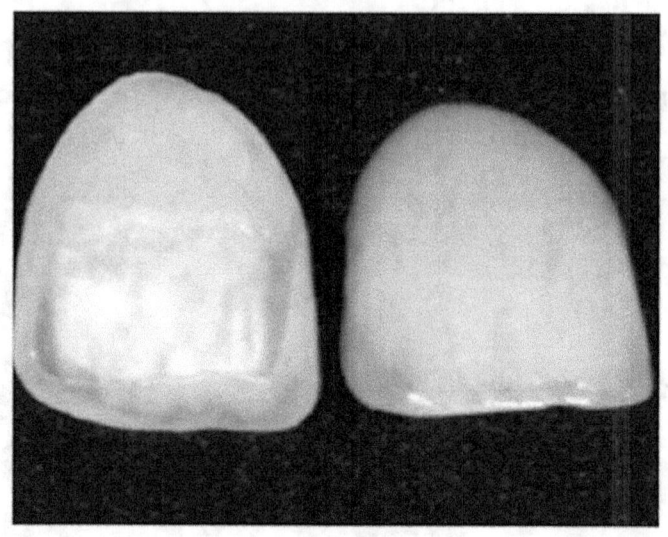

Porcelain Veneers

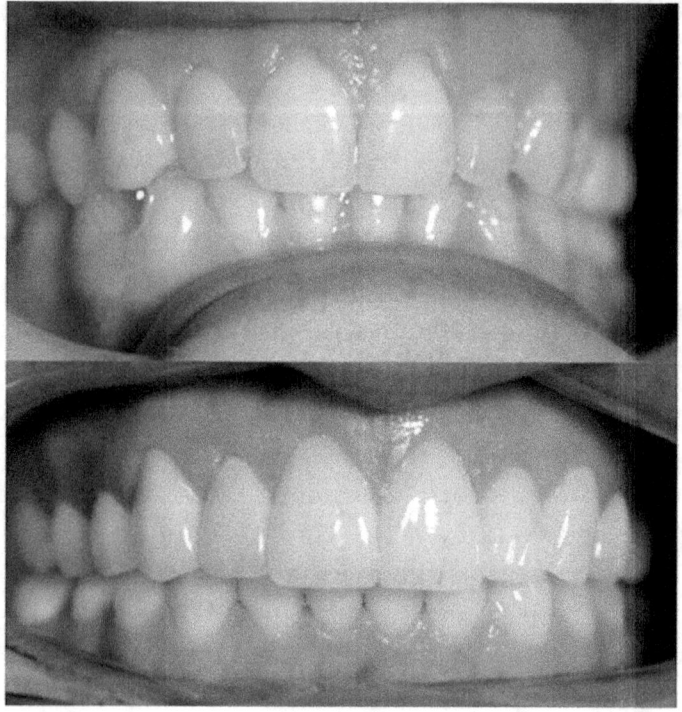

20 Porcelain Veneers

Dentists use veneers to accomplish restoration goals so that less tooth matter is removed. Some dental professionals believe that removing less tooth structure is more conservative and therefore healthier. Sometimes, it is actually more conservative to *remove* more tooth structure to protect a tooth over the long term if it means a crown or veneer will last longer.

In some cases, veneers cannot achieve all of the goals that the dentist has planned and a crown may be preferred. An example of this is in older patients, where the tooth structure isn't appropriate for bonding a veneer. As we age, our supporting dentin material becomes almost impossible to bond to. In these situations, crowns are the only way to reliably keep a tooth protected.

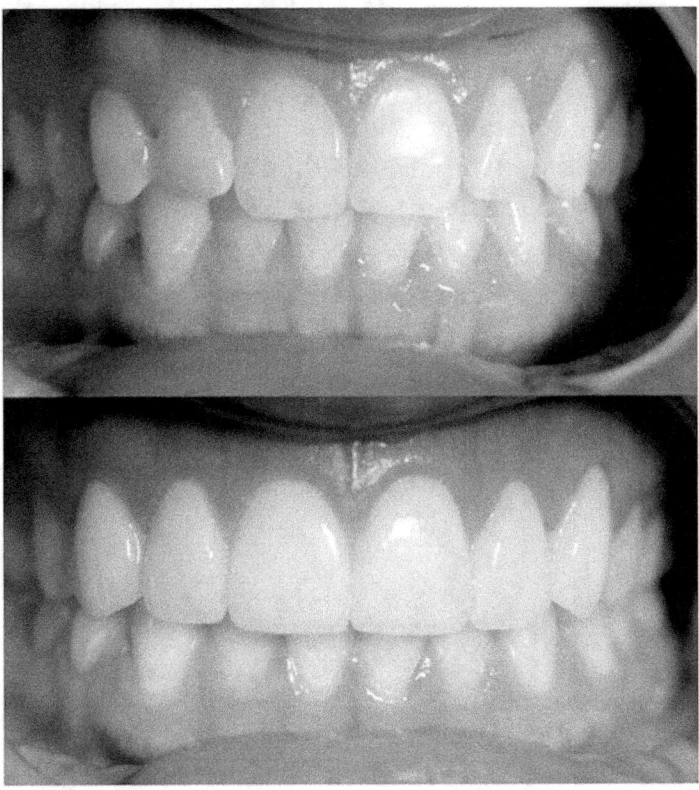

Veneers are always made of porcelain, while crowns can be made with metal under the porcelain for strength. Crowns in more cosmetic situations, such as on the front teeth are almost always all porcelain, while crowns on molars are usually metal and porcelain, providing more strength for heavier chewing.

You're a Supermodel

Zirconia is a white or oxidized metal that is becoming much more popular in dental restorations today. This material is as hard and strong as a typical metal, but is bright white and blocks out any dark colors in teeth. Studies show that zirconia is also extremely biocompatible and does very well in sensitive gum areas.

Zirconia is the material that I have chosen to use to create my Supermodel veneers and crowns with the help of my dental-laboratory owner, Dmitriy Taverdoff, CDT, of Dmitriy's Dental Studios. In the past, darker metals like gold and white gold were masked or blocked out visually with paint-like chemicals to make a tooth look white. This technique works, but requires more reduction of tooth structure to fit the material onto the restoration while retaining normal tooth size. Together, we have created a restoration that is beautiful, longer lasting, more biocompatible, and easily incorporated into cosmetic dental-restoration cases. My specific

preparation and the lab's unique material applications are a great combination when it comes to restoring teeth.

Crowns, implants, bonding, and veneers all work to modify the appearance, shade, and arrangement of teeth. These treatment modalities allow your dentist to design the smile of your dreams.

What to Look for When Choosing Your Cosmetic Dentist

There is no certified specialty program currently offered in North America for patients to find a great cosmetic dentist, although there are several associations that provide expert and hands-on training for dental professionals. There are some large training facilities that do a great job of educating their students in the art of cosmetic dentistry. Associations require dentists to submit cosmetic cases for credentialing and some private companies have educational programs that dentists can pay for to take different types of training. All training taken beyond dental school is effective and gives a dentist extra help when it comes to continuing education.

Different dentists have different ideas and levels of experience when it comes to cosmetic dentistry. You should always ask to see a dentist's own cosmetic work before you commit to sometimes-extensive treatment. Dentists should have a few really good examples of their own work on their website, so that you can be confident that you will obtain results with which you will be satisfied. Before and after photographs are also great ways for patients point out what type of look they want to achieve. For example, some patients may want the biggest, whitest teeth in the universe, while others may choose a more natural, translucent look.

Dental Laboratories

Dental labs come in all shapes and sizes, from small in-house dental-practice labs to huge full-service laboratories. The quality and caliber of their services can vary greatly and you don't always get what you pay for!

Labs will change in expertise over the years, as employment conditions change, meaning skilled technicians don't always stay at a lab long term, so it's good to know exactly which technicians will work on your case. Make sure that your dentist has a lab that he or she has worked with and is comfortable using. As with dentists, its OK to ask to see the cosmetic work their dental lab has done.

Try Before You Buy

What will my cosmetic makeover look like? Changing your smile is a major procedure. Most patients want to know what their teeth will look like after the procedure. One of the great things about cosmetic dentistry is that we have a few ways to "try before you buy."

The first way to see what your teeth will look like is to get something called a "cosmetic wax-up," which is a three-dimensional model of the outcome of your potential procedure that you can hold in your hand. It can be placed next to the original model—your current dental state—so that you can compare the before-and-after views of your teeth.

Some computer simulations can also be utilized. While I find that they can look nice, they are difficult for patients to really conceptualize what the image looks like in their own mouth. In my opinion, a physical model is preferable. I will often encourage patients to take home their models and show them to their support group and get input.

The third way patients can "try before they buy" is the creation mock-up done *in the mouth* of the post-procedural state. The cosmetic wax up can be used to make a "template" of a patient's new smile.

Dentists apply a tooth-colored plastic in the patient's mouth onto teeth without removing any tooth structure. I recommend this procedure only in dental cases involving eight to 10 teeth or more, or when a patient is apprehensive that the final outcome may not look good. The only situation that may affect this technique is one in which some natural tooth structure that needs to be removed by the procedure falls outside of the final contour of the cosmetic correction.

Using a cosmetic wax-up is much more useful after the teeth are prepared to receive cosmetic restorations, like veneers or crowns. The temporary restorations should be assessed a day or more after the procedure. Then, the patient returns to the dentist's office. Since the mouth is no longer numb, we can see how this new set of teeth will look, as well as assess speech and how much tooth structure shows in relation to the lips (assessment of the lip line). The "temporaries" are a close approximation of what the real teeth will look like after the procedure, but they can be altered or modified to make any desired changes. Once the final result is achieved, an impression is taken and a stone model is sent to the laboratory that fabricates porcelain restorations.

Lastly, composite or white filling material can be temporarily placed so that the patient can obtain a general idea of what their teeth can look like. This technique is best used in cases where the desired changes are minimal—as this can take hours—and needs to be done by a dentist or registered dental assistant.

The Ultimate "Try Before You Buy"

A patient usually tries on all restorations before their dentist cements them, so changes can be made if things are not ideal. Trying on permanent restorations is a time-consuming process, that's why we utilize cosmetic wax-up as a temporary restoration to see what the final outcome will look like.

What Is Your Perfect Smile?

Everyone is different and may want different dental outcomes! That's great. Your perfect smile is the one that makes *you* feel good about yourself. Maybe it's just a brighter and whiter smile. Maybe it's having some orthodontics to rearrange the way your teeth are aligned. It could even be getting some restorative work completed, such as crowns or veneers. Or most likely, it's a combination of a few different treatments.

There are numerous ways to improve your smile. This is *your* opportunity to take advantage of the new and exciting treatment options that have evolved from the dentistry of the past into Modern American Dentistry.

The smile of your dreams awaits you! And remember, **All Dentistry Is Cosmetic.**

Get ready for your own perfect smile!

Six ix porcelain crowns
Zoom whitening of lower teeth

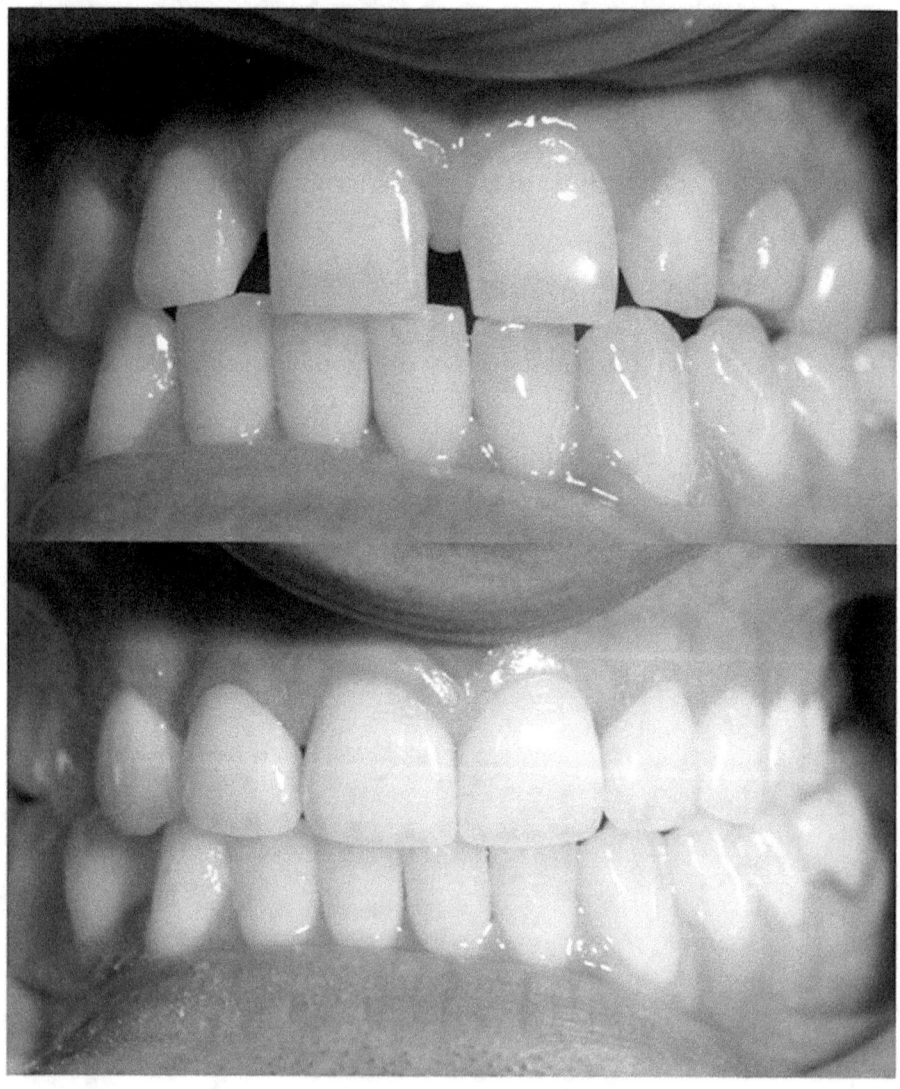

Six all ceramic veneers
whitening with opalessence

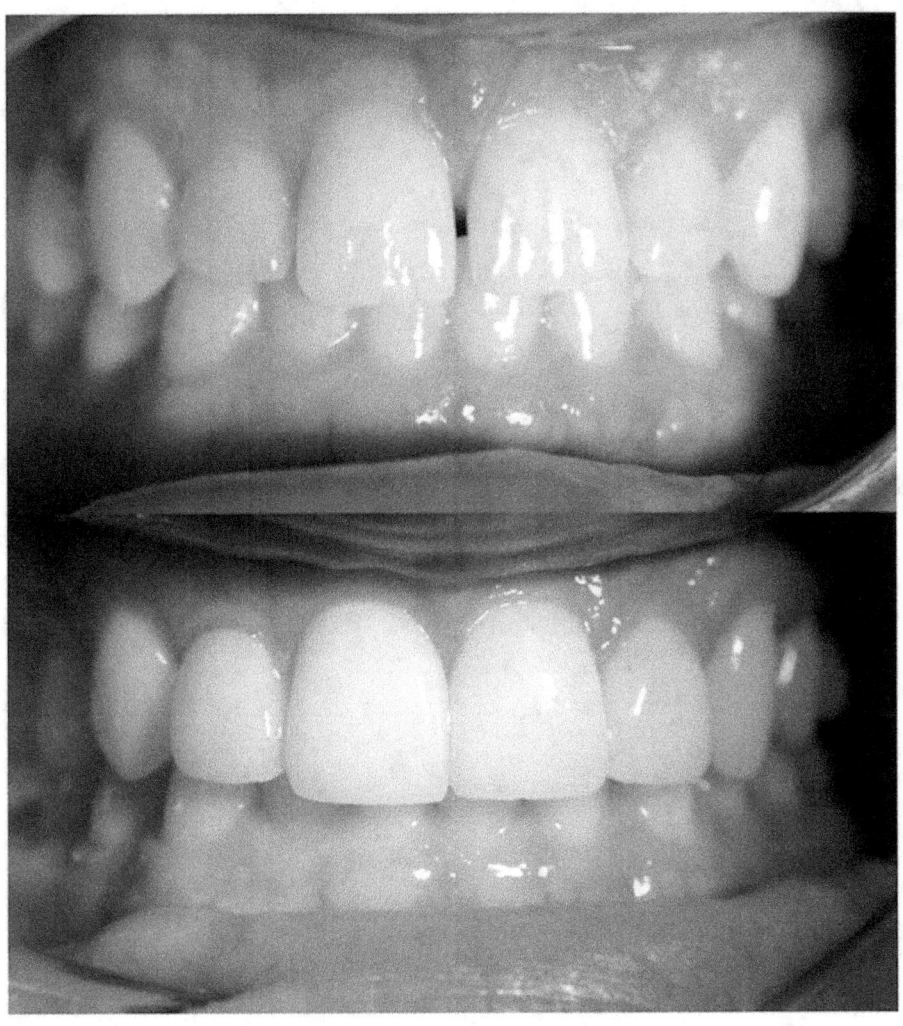

Six Super Model Veneers
Crest white strips for lower whitening

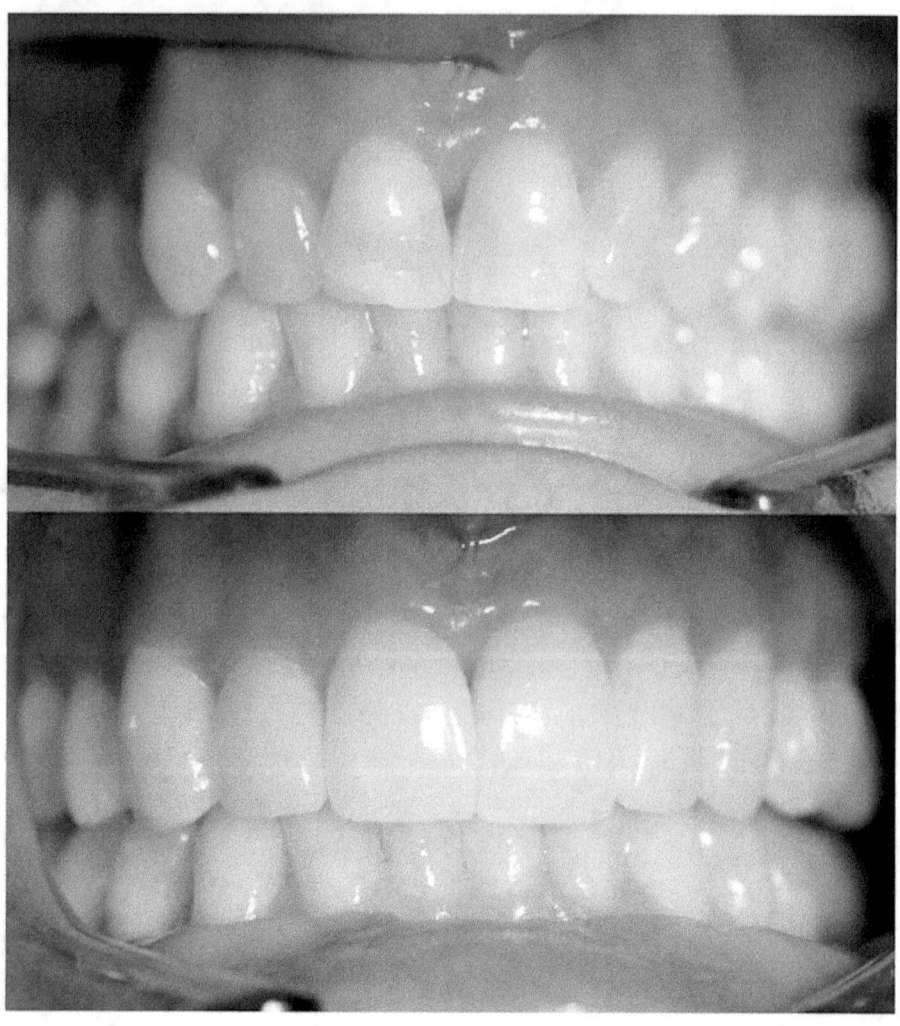

6 all Porcelain crowns
Opalessence Go!
Take home whitening

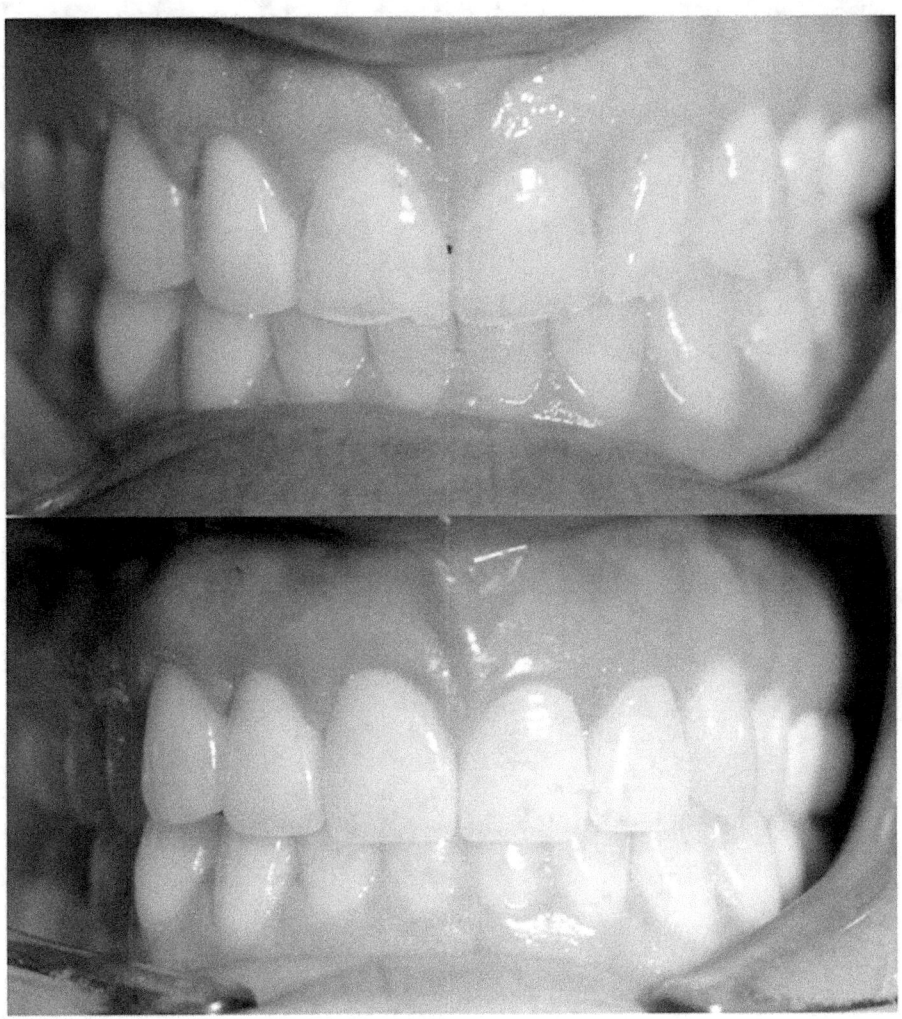

12 Supermodel Crowns

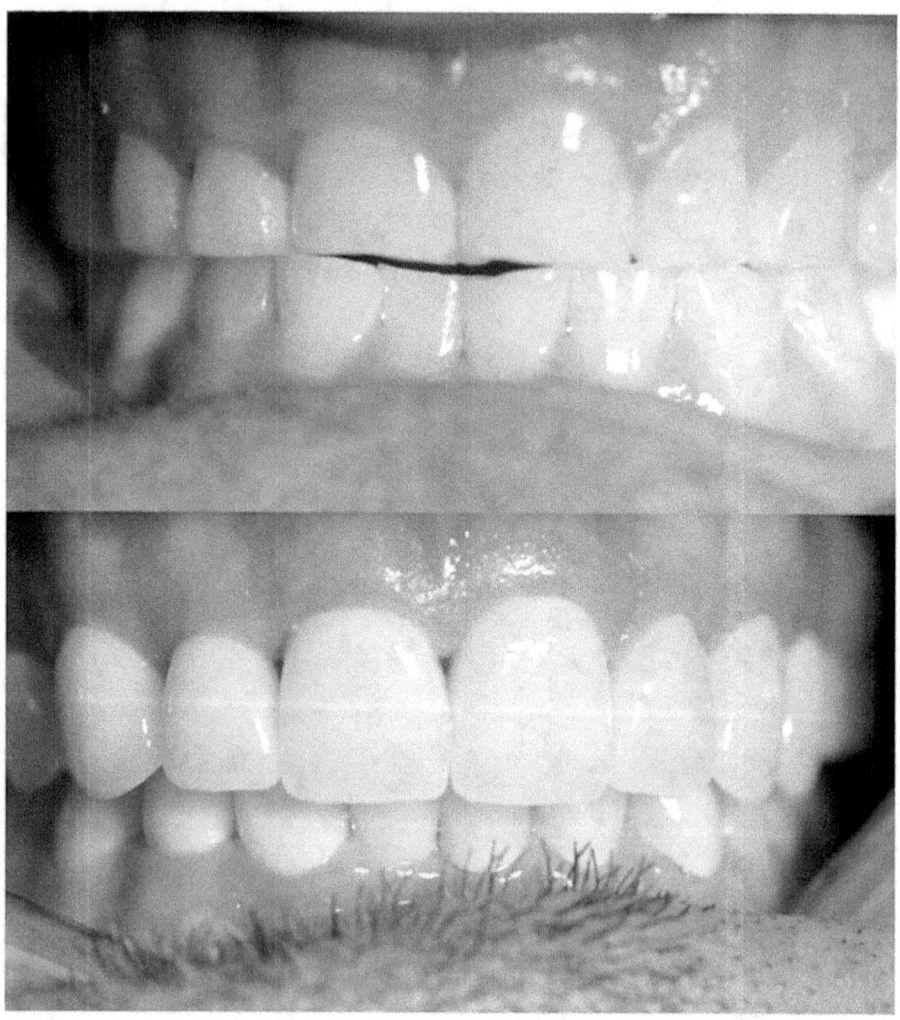

6 lumineers

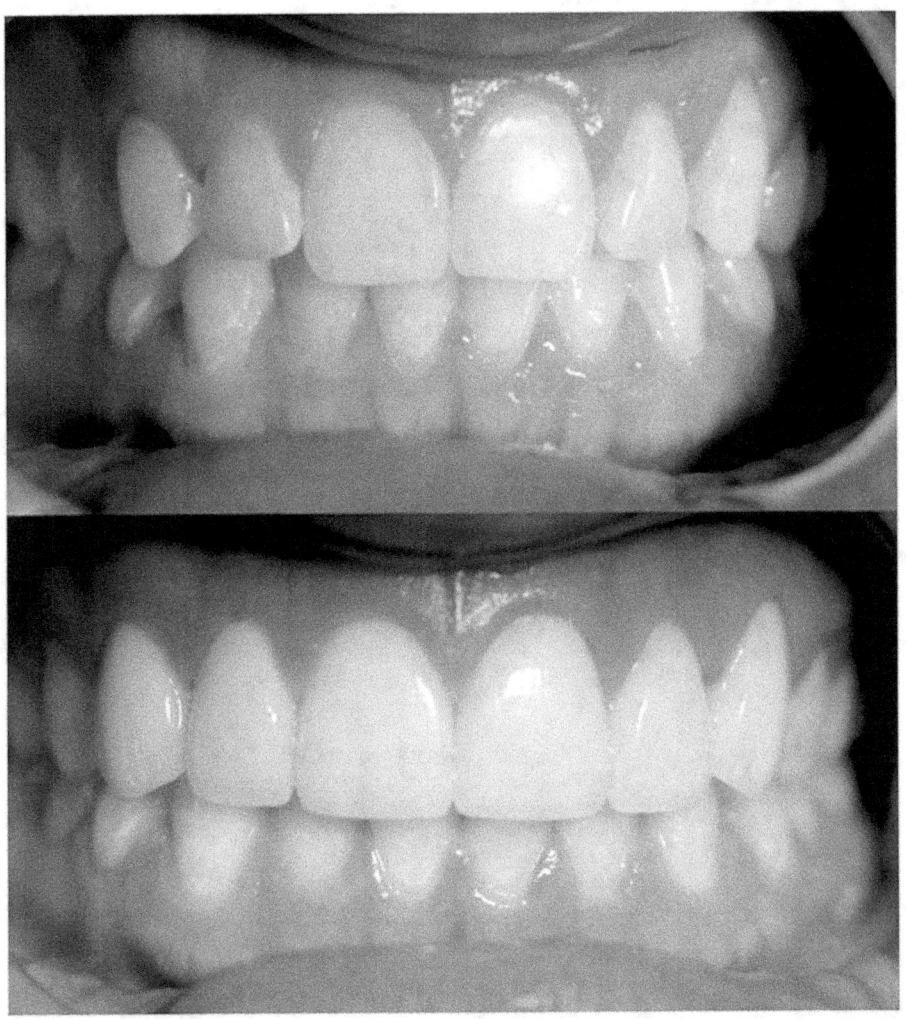

6 Super Model Veneers
Opalessence in office whitening

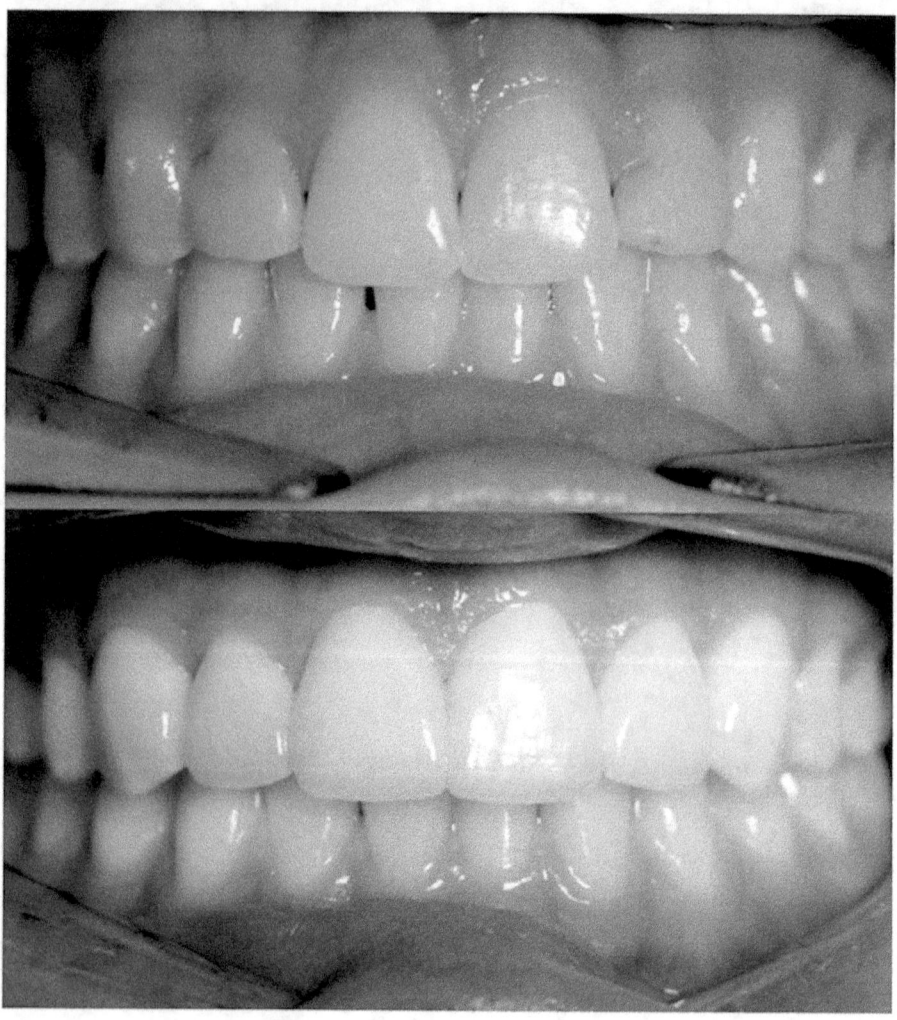

20 da Vinci veneers

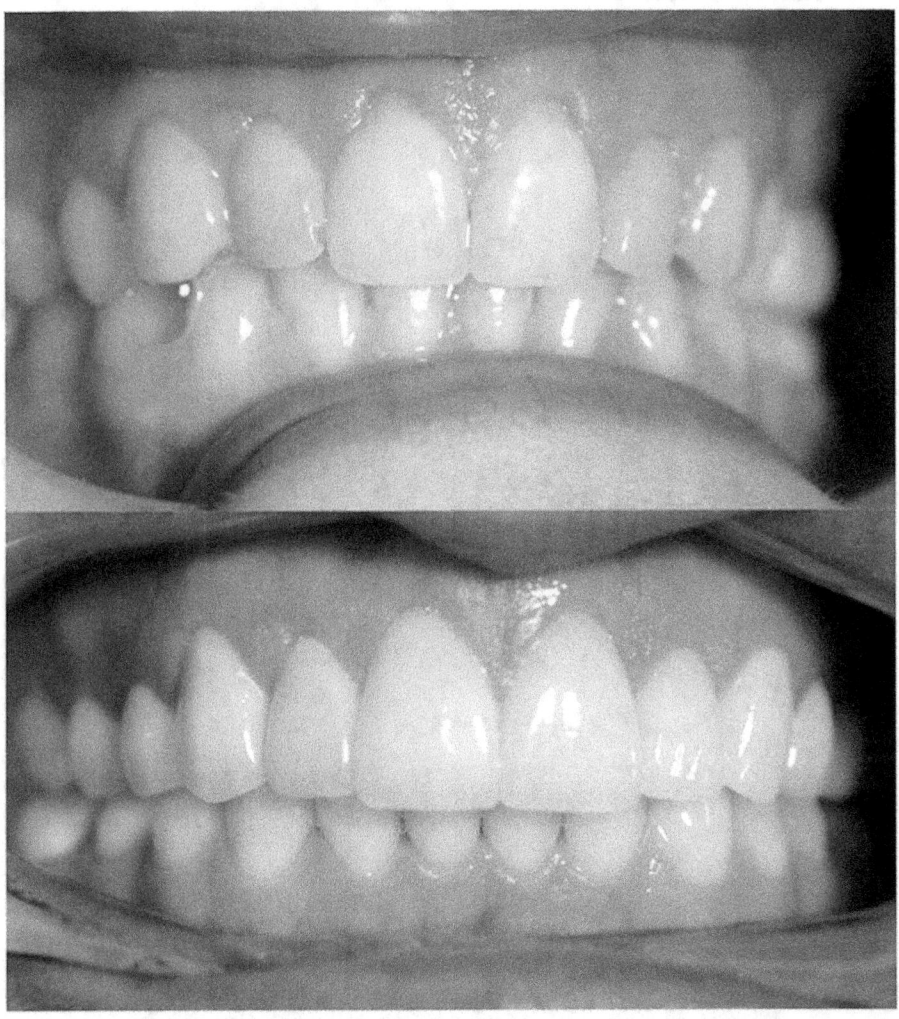

6 Super model Veneers
Micro Abrasion and Zoom whitening

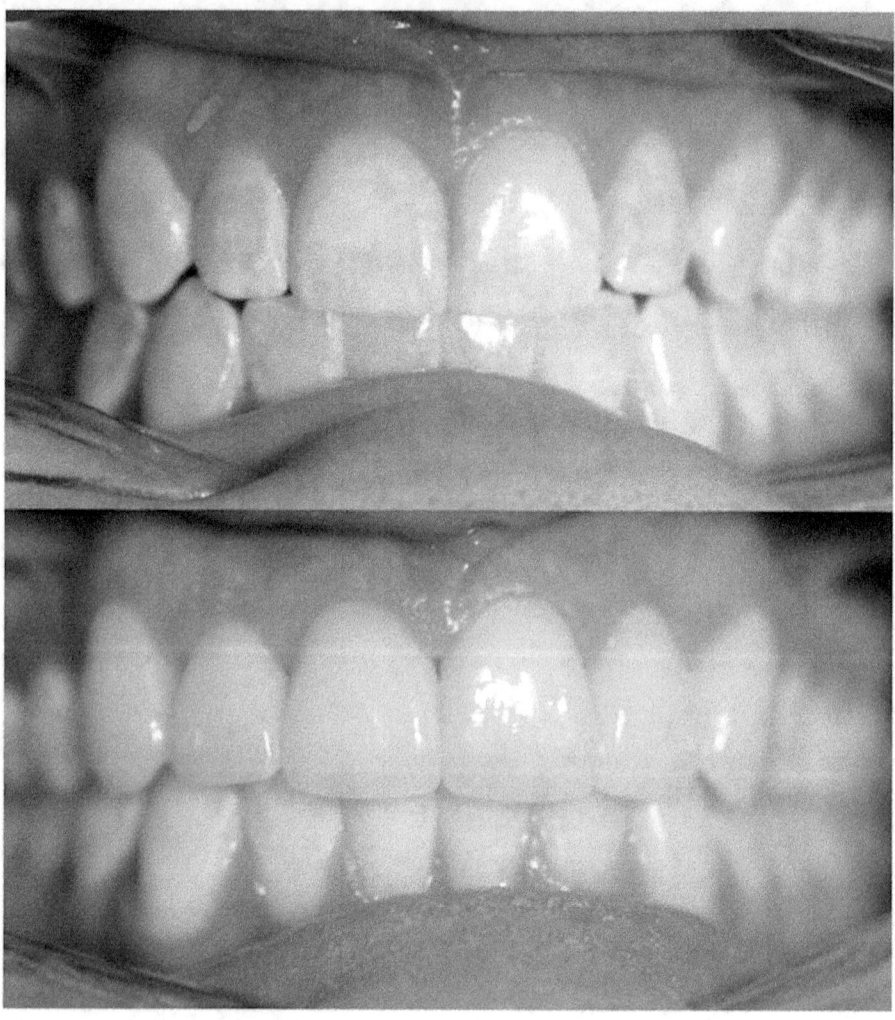

6 da vince Veneers

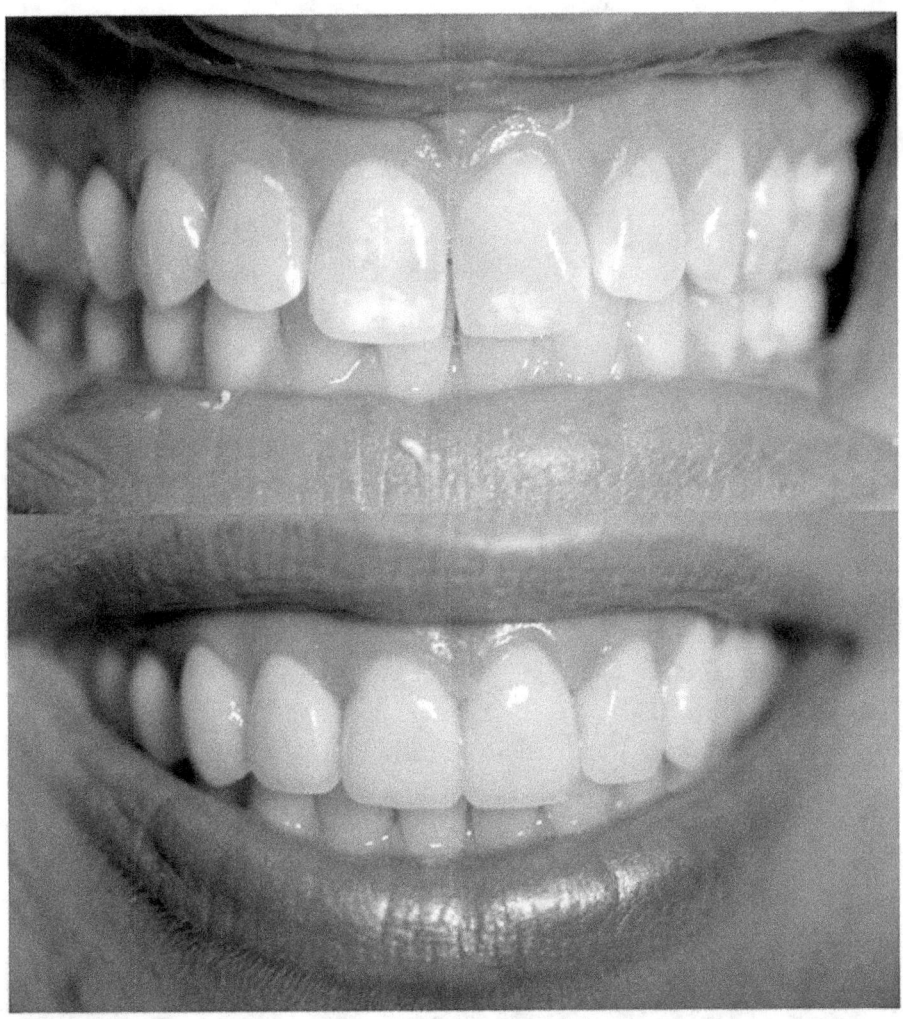

6 Super Model veneers
Crest White Strips

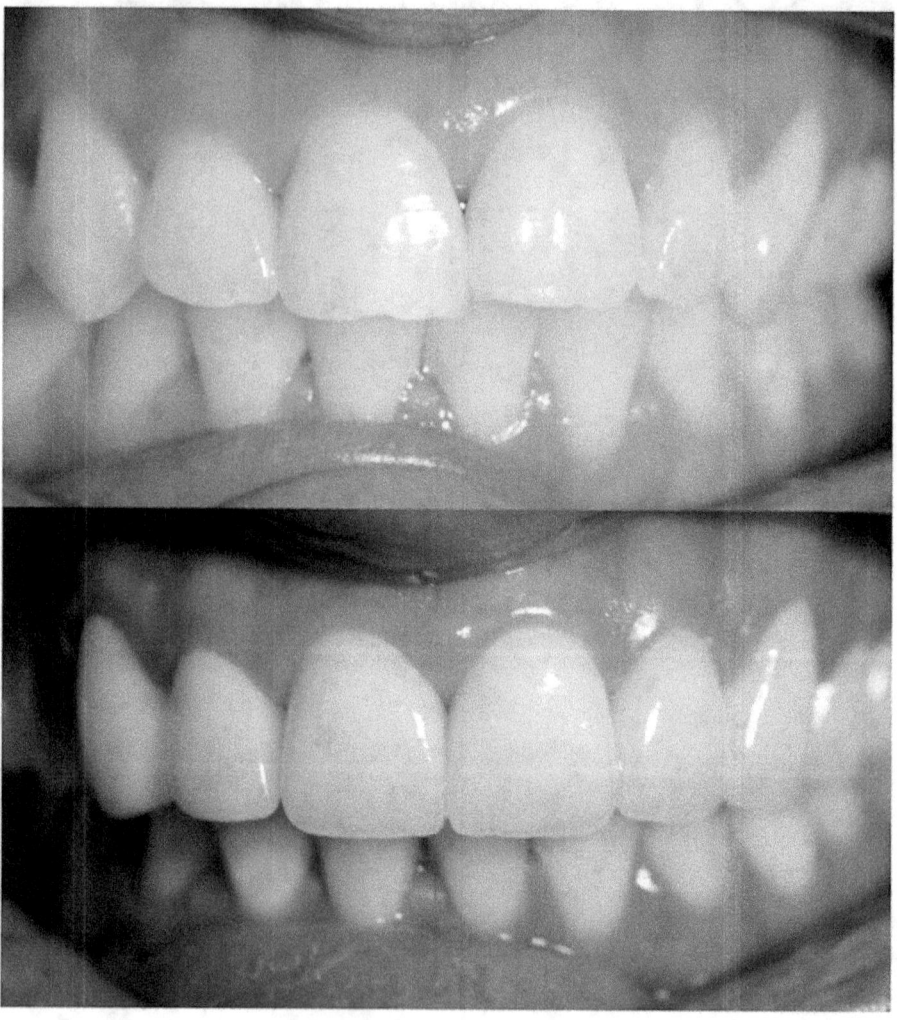

6 Super model Veneers
Oplaessence Whitening

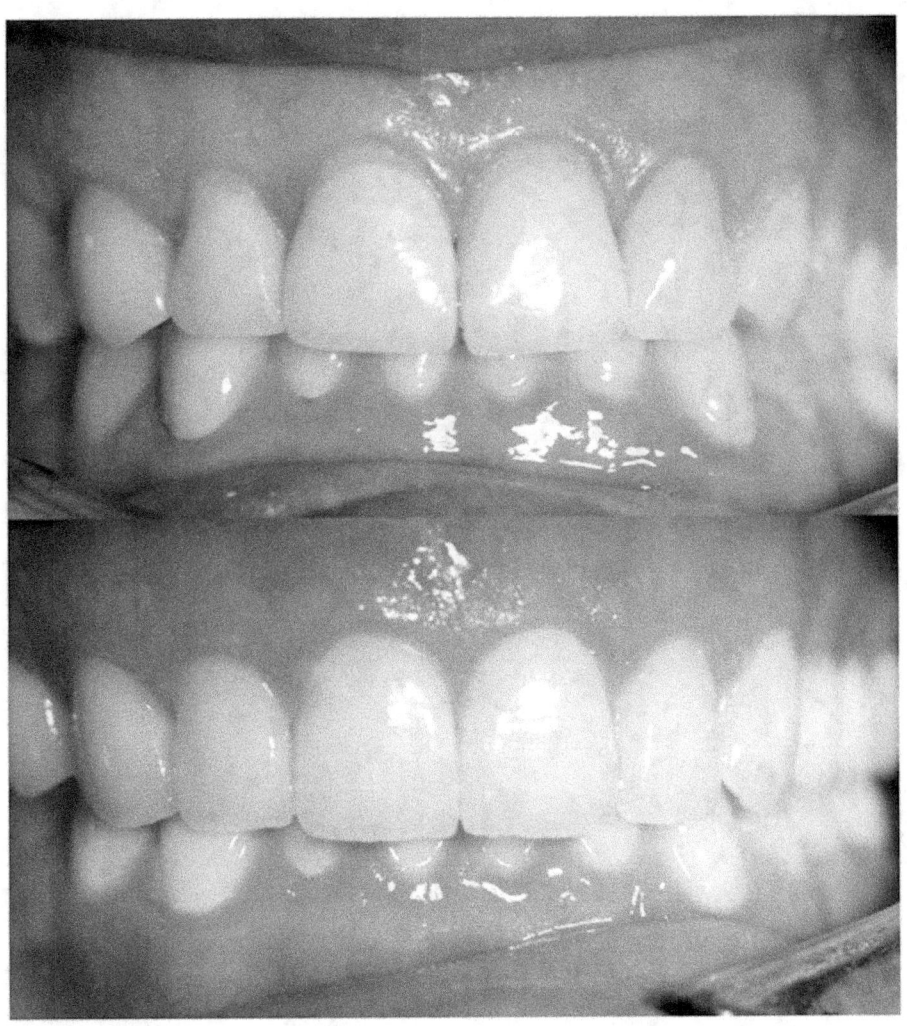

6 Super Model Crowns
Kor Whitening

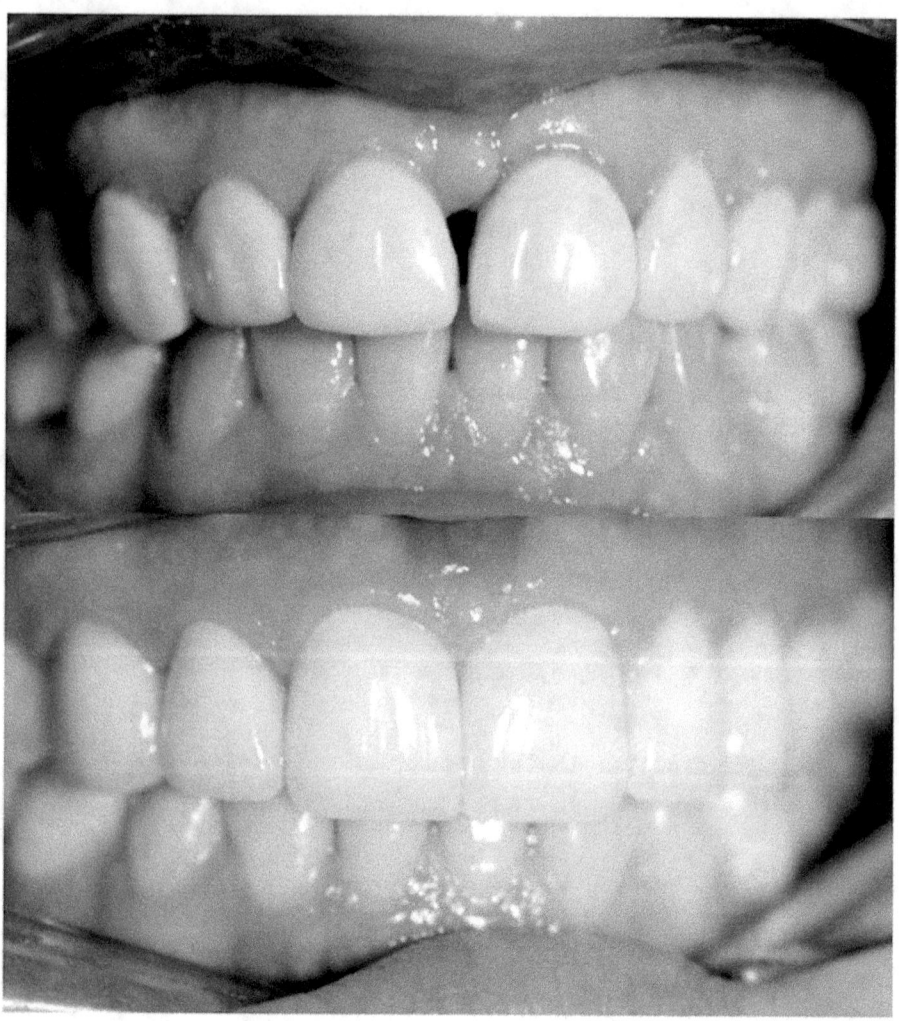

6 Da vinci Veneers
Zoom Whitening

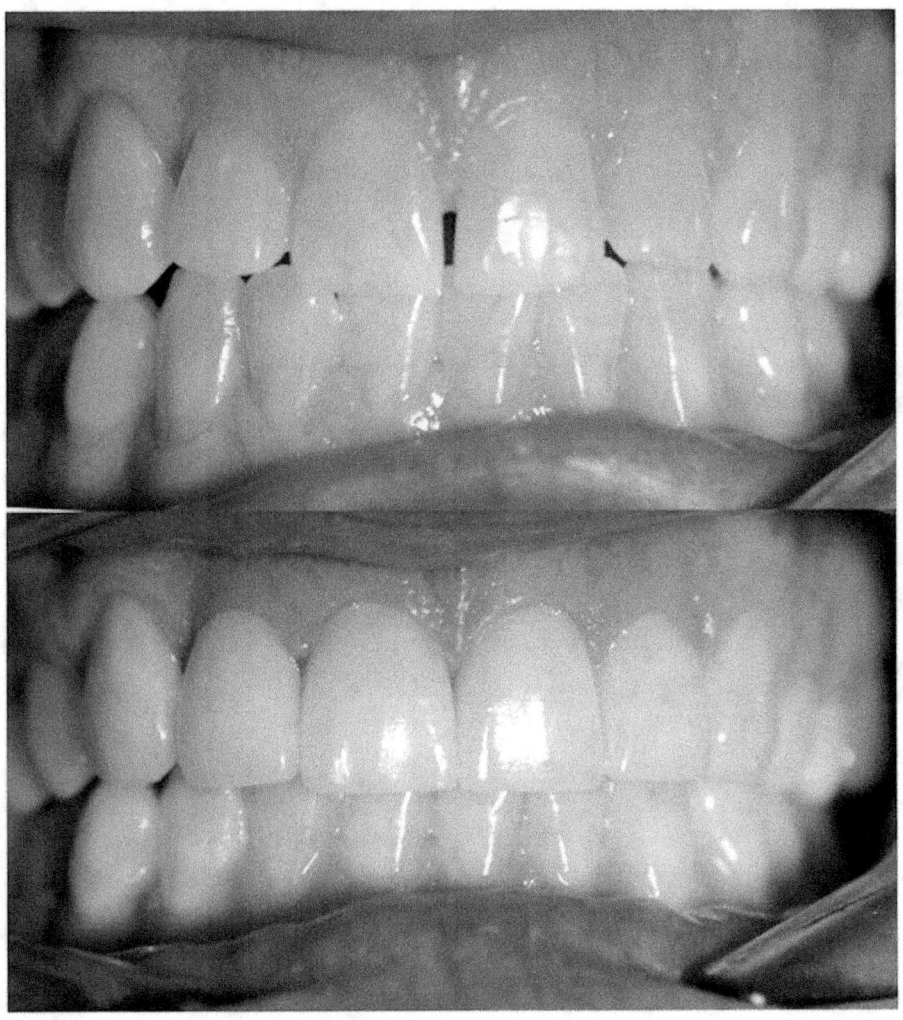

4 super Model Crowns
Opalessence whitening

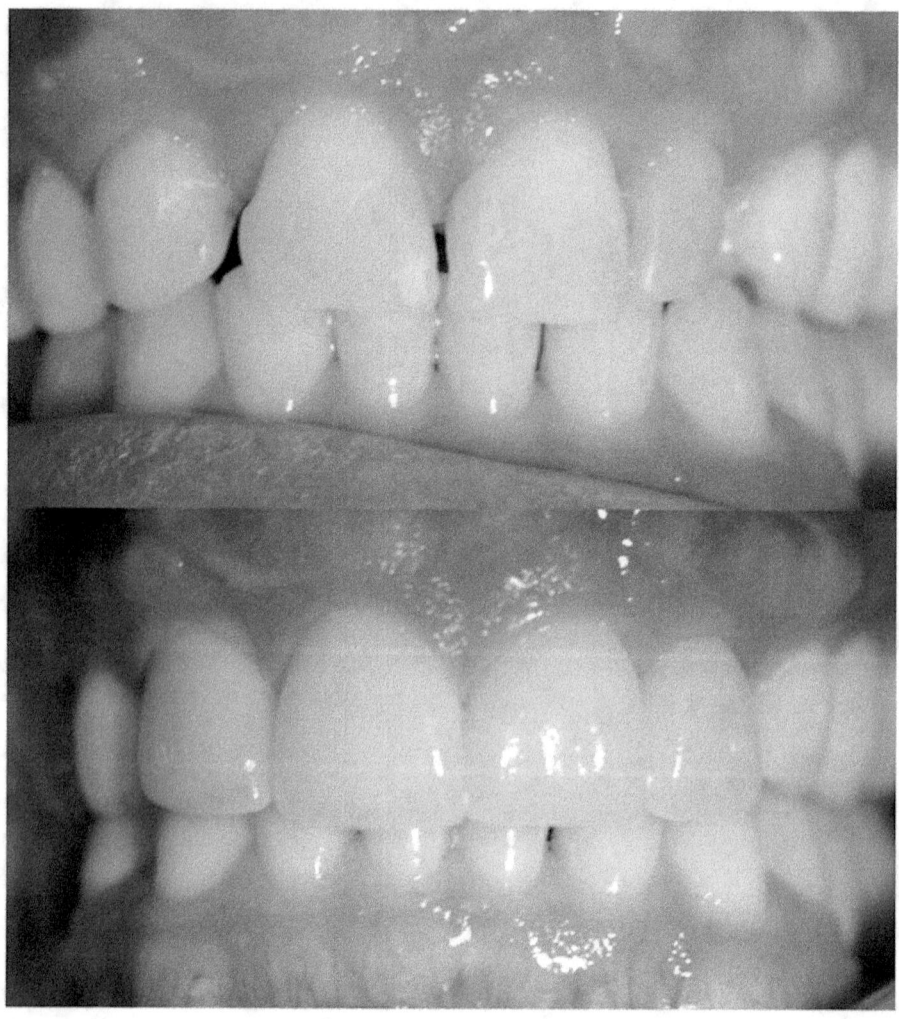

2 super Model crowns
2 super model veneers
Opalessence Go! Whitening

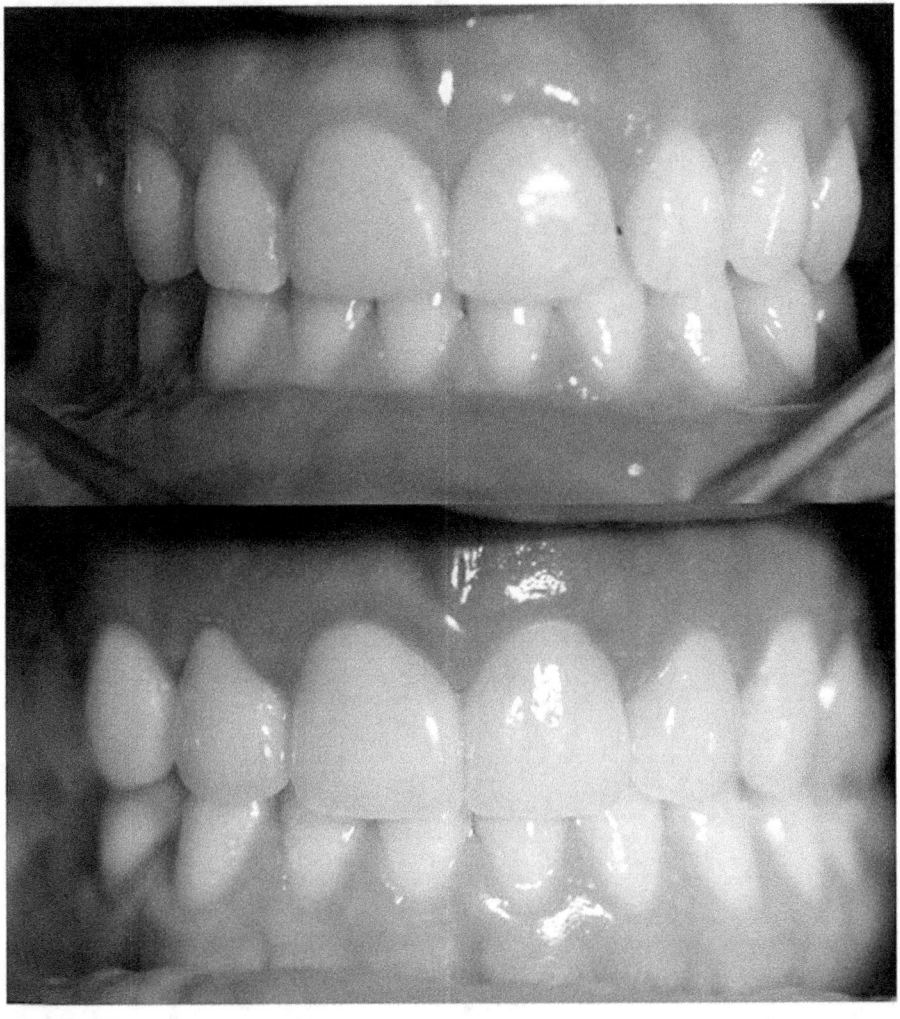

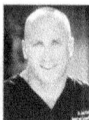

your look • the smile dr

By Dr. Joel Gould

Putting a
Cap on it

There's no capping your potential on the stage, runway, or screen, but the right dental work can make a huge difference in how you stand out

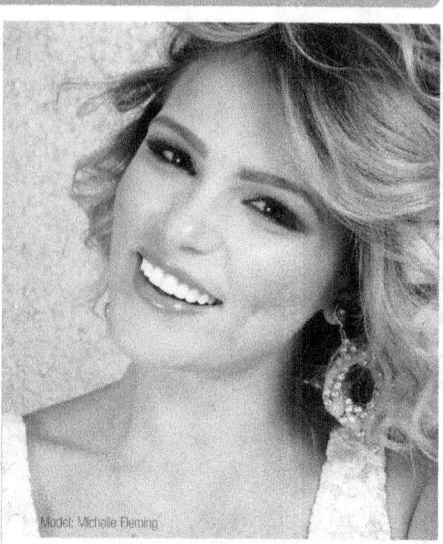

Model: Michelle Fleming

I n the glamour lifestyle industry, we have an expectation of an exceptionally beautiful, bright, perfect smile. While there are many beautiful smiles, such as Julia Roberts' unmistakable grin, nature isn't always so generous. It's great if you happened to win the genetic lottery and just naturally have the perfect smile. We see Hollywood actors and actresses such as Demi Moore and Sheryl Crow change their smiles right before our eyes with some very natural and stunningly beautiful veneers. Luckily, modern cosmetic dentistry allows anyone willing to invest the time and money into their mouths to also have a winning smile.

In my first article, I covered the elements of the perfect smile. Today I want to take you further. I want to take you behind the scenes of what a crown (AKA a cap) is, and how this differs from a veneer. Crowns and veneers are the main restorations dentists use to create the perfect smile.

The major difference between a crown and a veneer is the amount of tooth structure that is covered. Dentists choose a crown over a veneer for a patient when there isn't enough tooth structure to use a veneer. Veneers are most frequently used for cosmetic purposes only, but in certain situations, a veneer can also fortify a tooth, as well as make it look good. A crown is usually "cemented" in place, and some styles of crowns are also bonded, but veneers are always bonded in place. Bonding vs. cementation generally results in a much stronger connection between the restoration and the tooth structure.

A crown, or cap, is a dental laboratory-made restoration that is permanently cemented in place to restore and protect a tooth that has cracked, lost a large amount of natural tooth structure, or has had root canal treatment. Often-

times a crown is used to restore a tooth when a large filling fails and there isn't enough tooth structure left to support a new filling. Crowns are most frequently placed on back teeth, or molars. They can also be placed on front teeth to restore a damaged tooth to make it look brand new.

Crowns are used for both structural and cosmetic reasons. In today's hyper-fit world, we see our bodies aging relatively gracefully, however our teeth don't get the chance to regenerate at all. Once they erupt into the mouth they will remain unchanged until a dentist changes them. In fact, teeth and the cornea (the lens of the eye) are the only part of a human's body that doesn't regenerate millions of times throughout our lives.

A crown may be made of gold, porcelain, zirconia, or a combination of metal and porcelain (porcelain-fused to-metal or PFM crown). Zirconia is a relatively new material that is actually a metal (giving it unsurpassed strength) but in its oxide form exists as a white powder, giving it beauty. When choosing the right material(s) for a crown, your dentist must consider many factors, such as where in the mouth the crown will be placed, the types of forces the crown must withstand, whether or not the patient grinds or clenches their teeth, and if the crown will be used to support another dental device, such as a partial or a denture.

Crowns are prepared by the dentist by removing about a millimeter-and-a-half of tooth structure to allow for room to cover the entire tooth. An impression is taken and used by the lab to create a model and restoration. Newer impression materials taste better and set faster to make the ex-

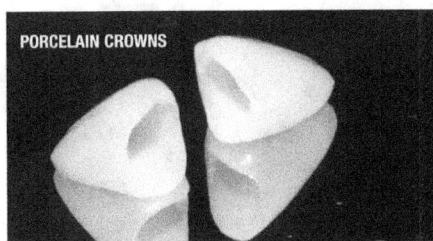

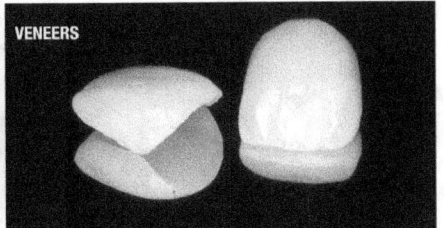

perience easy. You can think of a crown as a protective cap that completely surrounds the tooth, protecting it from damage, and restoring it to its former strength and beauty.

Veneers are commonly used in dentistry to improve one's smile. They can be used to correct misaligned, poorly-shaped and discolored teeth, and can drastically improve someone's smile in only a few visits. Teeth are prepared to receive the veneers by having anywhere between a half a millimeter, to several millimeters of enamel removed from the front and edge of the tooth. How much tooth structure is removed depends on what corrections are being made. This makes room for the porcelain veneer so that the finished product appears natural and not bulky.

Veneers are usually all porcelain. You can think of them in a similar way that imitation acrylic fingernails are bonded to your existing fingernails to make them look longer, uniform, ideal, polished and appealing.

Once a veneer is bonded to the tooth, it has about the same strength as a regular or natural tooth. Well-designed and properly-made veneers look completely natural, and can last for 25 years or more. Most need to be replaced after about 10 or 15 years due to gum recession, decay, or breakage. Aged veneers can easily be removed, and new veneers can be fabricated to change the smile back to its ideal.

There is no "one size fits all" or one specific technique in the field of dentistry. Procedures can vary greatly from one dentist to the next. Variables such as what part of the tooth and how much of it is removed can make a huge difference in the finished product. Also affecting the outcome is the use of different porcelains by the lab and the use of different cements by the dentist. We have seen many changes over the years as dentistry evolves, and the entire veneer experience is best in the hands of an experienced dentist. Actual before and after photos are a great way to see what your dentist and his dental lab can do, rather than seeing stock or generic photos. This may also give the patient an idea of the style of tooth she likes, and how her teeth could look.

Porcelain veneers are bonded to the teeth with a very strong adhesive. Depending on what outcome we are looking for, these adhesives can be tinted with different colors to try to match surrounding natural teeth. This process is very tricky, and it can be very difficult to match someone's natural shade. This is why we almost always do veneers in multiples and usually include at least the front upper or lower six teeth. This allows a uniform and symmetrical appearance that will look much more natural. When we are

doing an instant pageant makeover and creating the perfect smile, we usually veneer the top ten teeth. Each case is different and unique, and it's quite common to veneer all the way back to the first molars, again depending on how broad the smile is, and how far back teeth can be seen.

"Lumineers" are a brand name veneer. They are advertised as a reversible (or "no-preparation") veneer with very little removal of tooth structure. Lumineers are only about 0.2mm thick so they can be placed on top of your teeth without the removal of any enamel or tooth structure, therefore the procedure is reversible but has limited application.

Over the 25 years I have been practicing general and cosmetic dentistry, I have seen and placed many veneers, getting to know and understand how they age, and when and why they fail. The most common problems I see in failed veneers are deboning while eating, and gum recession that exposes the discoloration of the tooth that was previously covered by gum tissue. The "Supermodel Veneer" is a new type of veneer that I created with my dental laboratory, and its owner, Dimitriy Tarverdoff CDT of Dimitriy's Dental Studios in Los Angeles. I wanted to create a veneer that was bulletproof. I also wanted to simplify veneer placement, making them more predictable and, most importantly, longer lasting. This style of veneer is what I use for most of my larger pageant makeovers.

So to re-CAP (dental pun intended) dentists choose crowns or veneers, and sometimes both, depending on the individual needs of the patient. Veneers are made of porcelain, while crowns can be made from a combination of metal and porcelain. Both can be natural and beautiful, but ultimately it's the skill of the dentist, and the ability of the dental laboratory, that makes or breaks how natural cosmetic dentistry can look. □

Dr. Joel Gould has been practicing in Manhattan Beach since 2001. His general and cosmetic dental office treats patients of all ages and offers a broad range of treatments. Dr. Gould owned several practices in Vancouver, Canada for 10 years before moving to the Los Angeles area, and he has trained with several Beverly Hills plastic surgeons in the art and science of Botox and Juvederm. He collaborated with Dimitri's dental studios to create the "supermodel veneer" which he uses in his instant smile makeovers. Dr. Gould recently launched his new concept called "Modern American Dentistry," a no-nonsense approach to modern dental practice. With three locations, and five dentists, he has created a dental experience that is consistently comfortable.

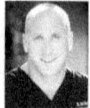

your look • the smile dr

By Dr. Joel Gould

An Unexpected End to Aches and Pains

While most people equate Botox with a wrinkle-free face, the popular treatment has been helpful in eliminating severe headaches

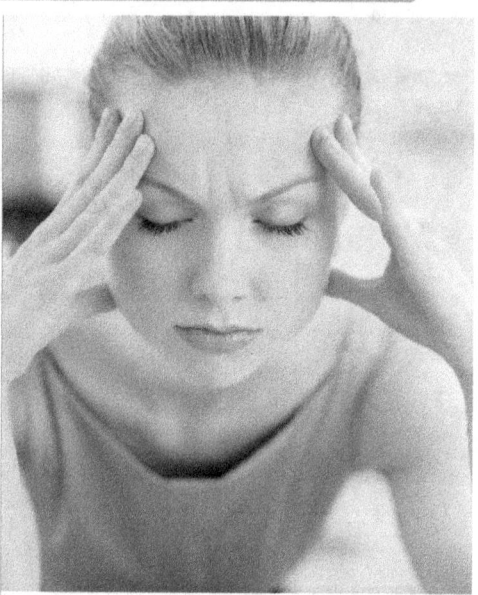

From the most glamorous stars in Hollywood who need to stay beautiful for the camera, like Oscar-winning actress Nicole Kidman and pop star Madonna, to average Americans who simply want to improve their appearances, Botox has enjoyed a wide embrace by the many medical practitioners who routinely use it on their patients with great success. Since its FDA approval and introduction to the public over a quarter-century ago, Botox has enabled millions of patients around the globe to reduce or eliminate both facial muscle conditions and cosmetic skin issues alike. Over 6 million Botox procedures are performed annually, making it the most common cosmetic operation today, keeping skin tight and smiles bright.

In recent years, Botox has been approved by the FDA to specifically help alleviate the pain of those who experience persistent and severe migraine headaches and muscle tension around the face, neck and head. This includes the temporomandibular joint, also called TMJ, which when overstimulated by stress, clenching and grinding, can also contribute to severe pain and tension headaches. The resultant pain is called Myofascial Pain Dysfunction Syndrome, or MFPD, *also* commonly referred to as TMJ. For some patients, Botox use has dramatically changed their lives, enabling them to resume dynamic activity, as well as the many other common experiences that most of us enjoy in good health.

But how does Botox work in these areas of the head and face? While medical leaders and researchers previously believed that severe headaches were driven by spasmodic blood vessels, many now understand that the high tension and repeated spasms of several flat muscle groups are responsible for migraines and TMJ. Botox causes partial muscle paralysis when injected locally to such tissues. It does this by dulling nerve endings that ordinarily trigger spasmodic muscle activity and it helps to interrupt recurrent pain cycles in patients.

Migraine headaches are those that occur to patients over half of the number of days in any given month. In addition to the severe pain in their head and face, sufferers often experience sustained feelings of nausea, as well as extreme sensitivities to light and sounds. There are a few different varieties of migraine headaches and, as such, some patients respond much better than others to Botox. Patients with migraines who feel that their face or head is being "squeezed" respond favorably to Botox, as well as those who experience facial muscle spasms or tension headaches. However, those with headaches between their eyes in the "orbit" area, those with headaches on the top of their head, on their cheeks or behind the ears have very little success with Botox.

A key area of the face that is amenable to Botox use is the upper mandible, where TMJ often occurs. As one of the most common orofacial pain sources for women and men, TMJ affects nearly a third of the population for those in their adult years. The causes of TMJ vary, though medical authorities believe it begins with indirect trauma or other psychological stressors. However, many patients have developed muscle or tendon disorders, which in combination with stressors, cause the symptoms of TMJ. Pain and tenderness where the upper jaw meets the temporal bone structure are often the first signs of TMJ, followed by limited use of or locking of the jaw, as well as repeated popping sounds that coincide with mandibular action during eating. The location of TMJ is crucial for its contribution to related migraines, myofascial pain and tooth pain. There, a collection of tendons, dense facial muscles and large nerve pathways intersect and extend outward. Often in TMJ, repeated subconscious clenching of the jaw or teeth, called bruxism, contributes to the problem.

Luckily, bruxism, migraines and TMJ have been greatly reduced by Botox use amongst patients. Doctors, dentists, facial plastic surgeons and trained medical personnel often administer Botox to their patients in several short sessions over time. Botox is injected with a small syringe in one of about four typical locations on the face or head. These include the temple region, the forehead, the inner orbital area near the eye or the upper region of the patient's neck. Depending on the acuity of the medical condition, anywhere from 4-10 injections of 2-5 units are administered to each area.

In many cases, patients are injected symmetrically, even if one side is the pain site, so that it does not switch to the opposing side of the face or head. Patients often improve greatly over the next few weeks or months. Botox is largely injected to the patient sites every three or so months to reduce the muscle tension that initiated their migraine and TMJ issues. It is an important goal to reduce the stressors that cause clenching and tension headaches; however, Botox allows the body to rest and repair, as well as not respond incessantly, which causes severe symptoms. This, in turn, enables patients to eventually reduce medication use and adjust behavior or destructive responses to stressors.

Despite FDA approval of Botox specifically for migraine headaches and other related maladies, many medical insurance companies do not cover the use of the medication. Often, a medical insurance company will require a patient to prove that his migraine has occurred over half of a year, for a majority of days in the month and for several hours every day. That same patient must have tried several other known prescription treatments for his condition. At that point, the neurologist must make a strong recommendation for the use of Botox in the patient's treatment. Only then can a patient qualify for insurance coverage of Botox use for migraines.

As Botox is derived from the neurotoxin and bacteria

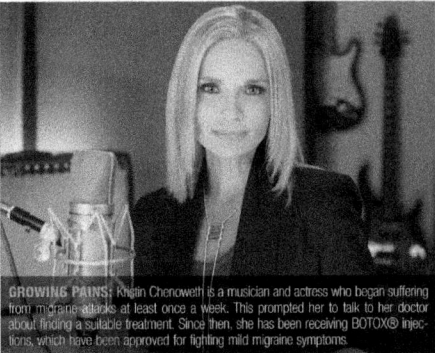

GROWING PAINS: Kristin Chenoweth is a musician and actress who began suffering from migraine attacks at least once a week. This prompted her to talk to her doctor about finding a suitable treatment. Since then, she has been receiving BOTOX® injections, which have been approved for fighting mild migraine symptoms.

known as botulism, it can cause some uncommon side effects. These include muscle paralysis and allergies. Some have encountered breathing issues, speech disorders, bruising, dry mouth, difficulty swallowing and others. A few deaths have been directly linked to Botox use, but none from cosmetic or migraine headache patients.

Many celebrities have, of course, used Botox for cosmetic purposes over the years with great effect. A few on the list of those who are open about their Botox use include television star Courteney Cox, Academy Award winner Gwyneth Paltrow, comedienne Jenny McCarthy, morning talk show host Kelly Ripa and supermodel Cindy Crawford, among others. Virginia Madsen, co-star of the award-winning feature motion picture *Sideways*, specifically used Botox to alleviate or reduce her recurrent migraine symptoms and stay beautiful, too.

Today, Botox has helped to reduce and prevent migraine headaches, facial pain and TMJ in millions of patients everywhere. The good news is that in the process, it also helps make facial wrinkles diminish and disappear, too. It's important to learn more about the dynamic benefits that Botox offers through qualified doctors or medical personnel who understand the practical applications of the medication and who use it regularly. With their help, migraine sufferers have been able to see the light at the end of the tunnel—and add a big helping of beauty in their lives. □

Dr. Joel Gould has been practicing in Manhattan Beach since 2001. His general and cosmetic dental office treats patients of all ages and offers a broad range of treatments. Dr. Gould owned several practices in Vancouver, Canada for 10 years before moving to the Los Angeles area, and he has trained with several Beverly Hills plastic surgeons in the art and science of Botox and Juvederm. He collaborated with Dimitri's dental studios to create the "supermodel veneer" which he uses in his instant smile makeovers. Dr. Gould recently launched his new concept called "Modern American Dentistry," a no-nonsense approach to modern dental practice. With three locations, and five dentists, he has created a dental experience that is consistently comfortable.

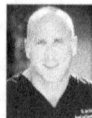

your look • the smile dr

By Dr. Joel Gould

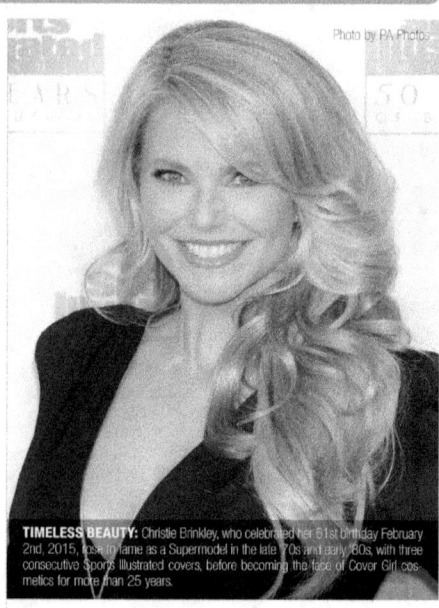

Photo by PA Photos

Your Face's Fountain of Youth

Dental anti-aging is a process that can help make your face look refreshed and young again, and it starts with your teeth

TIMELESS BEAUTY: Christie Brinkley, who celebrated her 61st birthday February 2nd, 2015, rose to fame as a Supermodel in the late '70s and early '80s, with three consecutive *Sports Illustrated* covers, before becoming the face of Cover Girl cosmetics for more than 25 years.

Time marches on, constant and unforgiving! How do celebrities look so young? Christie Brinkley, Jennifer Aniston, Halle Berry, all seemingly remain young and beautiful. Sure, a line of cosmetics is a great side business for Cindy Crawford, but is that really all she is doing?

Dentistry has come a very long way over the years. There was a time that it was normal and expected that as adults aged, they would eventually lose all of their teeth, and be destined to wear dentures for the rest of their lives. Thankfully, modern science and medicine have evolved and given us myriad sophisticated dentofacial treatments to turn back the clock, and reverse the normal course of aging.

The main objective of Anti-Aging Dentistry is to focus on prevention of loss of natural facial structures that result in the appearance of aging, and to restore the lower face to a more youthful iteration by utilizing all of the latest aspects of Medicine Dentistry and Facial Esthetics.

As a healthcare provider, I strongly advocate for a balanced healthy lifestyle. Oral health is conclusively linked to Alzheimer's disease, as well as diabetes and even heart disease, as if you didn't need another reason to floss!

Experts unanimously recommend a diet rich in unprocessed foods, with plenty of healthy fruits and vegetables, which, in addition to drinking plenty of water, will help keep you hydrated due to their fiber content. (Avoid the killer fruits and veggies, such as potatoes and papayas.) Regular exercise will also go a long way to keep you looking young. Exercise, especially frequent cardiovascular and muscle building activity, has been proven to increase pro-

duction of healthy hormones such as the recently highly touted "Human Growth Hormone" or HGH.

Our own natural production of HGH depressingly peaks at about age 17, and then gradually fades, rapidly at first as we age. HGH is a large molecule similar to estrogen and testosterone that humans produce naturally in our pituitary gland (deep in our brainstems) and is released into the bloodstream where it reaches all tissues, and interacts in many ways to keep us younger, and make us healthier.

HGH is a virtual fountain of youth, proven to reduce body fat, increase lean muscle mass, elevate mood, strengthen bones, boost libido, support our immune system, speed healing and reduce wrinkles by rejuvenating our skin. Synthetic HGH has been used for years by professional athletes, as well as Hollywood superstars. Science shows us that its use, while effective, may alter pituitary function, and its long term effects are still unknown.

There has been a huge push towards HGH precursors, or antecedents. Several companies have proven data, showing increases of up to 600 percent in natural HGH production, by our own pituitary glands; meaning that by supplying the building blocks of this wonder molecule in large amounts, our bodies actually produce a significantly elevated level of circulating HGH in our bloodstreams.

By taking these building blocks of HGH in specially-

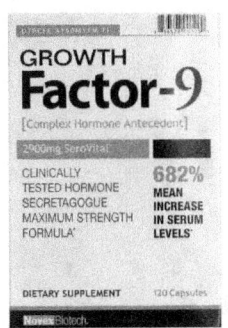

GROWTH
Factor-9
[Complex Hormone Antecedent]

2900mg SeroVital

CLINICALLY
TESTED HORMONE   **682%**
SECRETAGOGUE   MEAN
MAXIMUM STRENGTH   INCREASE
FORMULA'   IN SERUM
     LEVELS'

DIETARY SUPPLEMENT   120 Capsules

Novex Biotech.

FOUNTAIN OF YOUTH: Scientists have developed an oral formula that encourages the pituitary gland to increase growth hormone production at a more youthful rate.

coated capsules, two hours after eating, and not eating for another two hours after ingestion, they are able to travel to the right area of the small intestine to be efficiently absorbed for maximum uptake into the blood stream, without being destroyed by our stomach's acids.

This new development may alter who we are as a people, by allowing us to turn back the clock so significantly, that we may need to rethink our dreams of extensive life longevity. There are very few studies that can show us what this increased level of HGH may do, and it may take us many years to discover its unknown and unintended consequences, beneficial or harmful.

Periodontal or gum disease is a chronic low grade infection that results in a change in bacterial growth, ultimately causing inflammation of the gums (Gingivae)—with associated bleeding, and loss of bone in the mouth, often leading to the loss of teeth. Decay (dental decay and cavities, also known as "Dental Caries") is a bacterial infection of one or more teeth, leading to loss of tooth structure, and subsequent infection of the dental nerve, or pulp, and abscess formation.

These two villains of oral health are the major cause of deterioration of the oral cavity, and surrounding structures, preventing their effects will arrest aging completely. Furthermore, reparative dental procedures will reverse aging and restore the mouth to close to pristine condition.

Effective regular preventive care, consisting of cleaning, deep cleaning, and in some cases even surgical intervention will prevent gum disease from eroding bone around the mouth. Beautiful, protective, and functional dental restorations such as crowns, veneers, and implant bridges can bring a broken down smile back to life, focusing on proper cheek and lip support, color, shape, and arrangement for a youthful smile. Unsightly gum recession, causing roots to be exposed and look aged can now be successfully covered by a new gum surgery technique called the "Chao Pinhole surgical technique," which is a huge improvement from the older, more painful gum grafts from the roof of the mouth.

We utilize orthodontics more these days due to revolutionary clear aligner systems, such as Invisalign, which moves teeth gradually into the ideal positon through a series of custom clear trays, worn 22 hours a day, and changed out every two weeks. Aligned teeth wear better and more evenly, preventing excessive and unsightly wear patterns, and the destruction of natural tooth shape.

Today's hyper-stressed world has caused many of us to find that we are heavy clenchers, or grinders, and we are putting a tremendous force on our teeth and jaws. Dentistry can offer several different designs of "Bruxguards" or mouth guards that will allow tired muscles to relax, and insulate teeth from uneven wear due to excessive clenching and grinding. This phenomenon, often called TMJ, can have devastating effects on the youthfulness of our smiles.

To restore facial youth, gradual layering of dermal fillers such as Juvéderm using an amazing new technique called "Blunt Tip Cannula" (a thin, long flexible needle with a blunt end that we have happily renamed "Bruise-free Facial Filler" or "BFF") keeps facial tissues firm, plump, and youthful. This procedure can be done on your lunch break, and you can return to work immediately, with little to no pain, and almost no bruising or swelling.

Traditional dermal filler techniques with a regular needle can cause pain, severe reversible swelling, and bruising. Applied correctly, these safe clear viscus gels consisting of Hyaluronic acid can replace the fat, stimulate collagen production, and reform and rejuvenate lip shape that may have been lost over the years, including smoker's lines. Synthetic collagen, as well as one's own fat, can also be injected into the face to prevent a tired and sunken look. These procedures are routinely done by plastic surgeons, and can be successful. Fillers are best placed gradually over time, and will significantly hold off wrinkling, and aging skin appearance. I advocate placing these fillers early, so that facial volume will not be lost, although when strategically placed, it can almost completely restore an aging face to a youthful state.

Botox, a purified protein proven to reduce wrinkles, can be used around the eyes (crow's feet), the "number 11's" between the eyes (Glabellar muscle, also called frown lines), and across the forehead (Frontalis muscle) will slightly lift eyebrows, and can reduce migraines to give a more refreshed look to the entire face. I find most of my patients are shocked that Botox can enhance someone's appearance, giving them a refreshed look, without making them look weird.

Sure, celebrities look like they are staying young, and while we can't stop time, we can slow it down. With prevention and proper use of procedures and techniques, there is no need to be long in the tooth, with the help of all of today's exciting advances, we can greatly diminish its effects on our faces and psyche. □

Dr. Joel Gould has been practicing in Manhattan Beach since 2001. His general and cosmetic dental office treats patients of all ages and offers a broad range of treatments. Dr. Gould owned several practices in Vancouver, Canada for 10 years before moving to the Los Angeles area, and he has trained with several Beverly Hills plastic surgeons in the art and science of Botox and Juvederm. He collaborated with Dimitri's dental studios to create the "supermodel veneer" which he uses in his instant smile makeovers. Dr. Gould recently launched his new concept called "Modern American Dentistry," a no-nonsense approach to modern dental practice. With three locations, and five dentists, he has created a dental experience that is consistently comfortable.

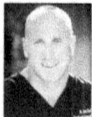

your look • the smile dr

By Dr. Joel Gould

Instant Smile
Makeover

In understanding the elements of a winning smile, anyone can utilize today's best dental and cosmetic techniques in getting a head start on the competition

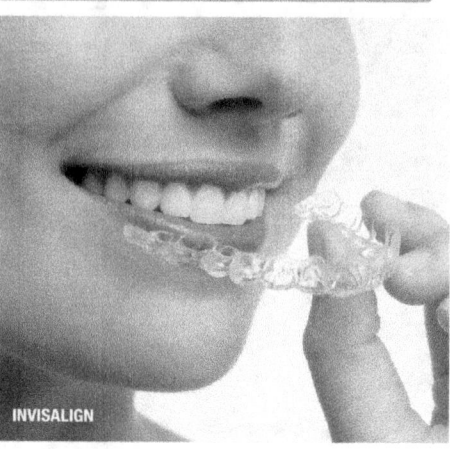

INVISALIGN

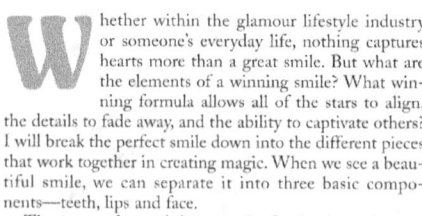

W hether within the glamour lifestyle industry or someone's everyday life, nothing captures hearts more than a great smile. But what are the elements of a winning smile? What winning formula allows all of the stars to align, the details to fade away, and the ability to captivate others? I will break the perfect smile down into the different pieces that work together in creating magic. When we see a beautiful smile, we can separate it into three basic components—teeth, lips and face.

The eyes and mouth become the focal points when we notice someone with a winning smile. Full, defined youthful lips frame naturally-shaped teeth with translucent white color, just as the eyes are surrounded by a smooth, youthful textured skin, with the eyebrows preferably slightly-arched. All of these elements can be enhanced by a qualified and talented dentist, trained in natural-looking dentofacial esthetics. Let's focus on teeth and lips, as we zero in on a radiant smile that can light up a room and impress at a competition.

SETTING THE RIGHT ARRANGEMENT

Orthodontists are dental specialists that are trained in the arrangement of teeth. New techniques for straightening teeth have evolved, and inventions such as Invisalign and other clear aligners are an exciting change to those old metal railroad tracks that were anything but beautiful. Clear aligners are thin plastic trays, custom fabricated by a high tech computer program and changed every two weeks, and are barely visible. They should be worn for at least 22 hours a day, but are easily removed for meals, and any important social functions.

These trays make small changes as teeth move to the

ideal alignment desired. With tooth-colored brackets and "lingual braces" (brackets on the inside of teeth, so they are invisible) it's easy to change an average smile into a wow-factor smile.

When there is more than one issue with a tooth, dentists often turn to veneers, or all porcelain crowns. In addition, dentists may use dental implants and tooth-colored fillings to be able to provide a great-looking smile.

LOOKING WHITE IN THE TOOTH

With cosmetic dentistry and white teeth visible in every well-photographed model's smile, the industry has risen to the occasion, with a large variety of over-the-counter, take home and do-it-yourself tooth whitening systems. Zoom!, Opalessense and Brightsmile are well-known, in-office one-hour tooth whitening systems, found to be safe and effective for a relatively permanent color change.

With any tooth-whitening, the results can be prolonged by using a Sonicare or similar electric-style toothbrush, and the vibrations of the brush will help to prolong the improved shade over time. Cutting down on red wine and other darkly-pigmented foods may be a bit boring, but it will keep your smile brighter, longer.

BELIEVE IN VENEERS

Veneers, or porcelain veneers as they are called, are porcelain facings that are literally bonded to the front of an existing tooth that can change the color, shape, size and arrangement instantly. These restorations are durable and can look completely natural when the dentist collaborates with a talented laboratory, as the makeover effect can be shockingly dramatic and spectacular. Discolorations, chipped and misaligned or rotated teeth can be instantly

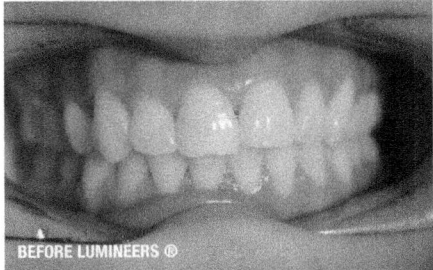

BEFORE LUMINEERS ®

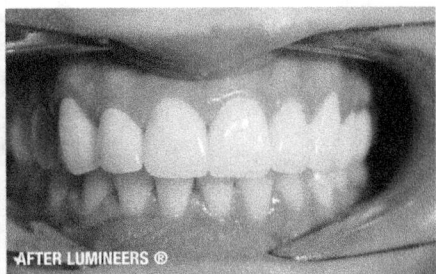

AFTER LUMINEERS ®

transformed to a set of ideal pearly whites. This is instant gratification at its best, as the results are visible at the first visit. When it comes to how many veneers are needed for a true smile makeover, we need to take into account how big of a smile our subject projects to achieve our ultimate goal. A winning smile usually exposes teeth all the way back to the first molar, and the dentist and patient can decide whether we need to change six, 10, or even 20 teeth to achieve an ideal instant smile makeover.

Lumineers and the supermodel veneer are two different brands or styles of veneers that are utilized by dentists. Different porcelains are fabricated and designed to specifically suit the patient's specific needs.

The different elements of the face, lips and teeth can be brought together by a great cosmetic dentist. With modern technology, and an experienced dental team, anyone can have the winning smile of their dreams.

FACING THE FILLER FACTS

Some dentists treat their patients with Botox and dermal fillers such as Juvederm. As doctors of the mouth and associated structures, a dentist can be trained and highly skilled at these injections, and after all, who gives more shots than dentists? These medications can be used to diminish facial lines and give areas of the face a firm and youthful look.

GIVING SOME LIP

Lip augmentation techniques used to achieve cosmetic improvements vary greatly from provider to provider, based on their training, experience and artistic talent. Dentists can utilize their knowledge and understanding of how the lips rest on the teeth. They use specific dental measurements to be able to create a very natural smile, while avoiding the pitfalls of many inexperienced injectors creating a trout pout or duck lips.

Different products are available to use in the face and lips and are called "dermal fillers." You may have heard of two of the more popular brand names, Restalyn or Juvederm. They contain a substance called hyaluronic acid, which is a clear, purified viscous gel that is hypoallergenic. As we age, women especially will lose their own natural hyaluronic acids. Fine and increasingly deeper lines can be filled comfortably with these products. Dentists can use Novocain to numb the lips and avoid pain that can sometimes be intense

during the injections. As these products often last more than six months, the dental office can be an ideal place to maintain a youthful appearance, with both ease and comfort.

Lip augmentation should be highly-customized to suit a person's face, as a set of "one size fits all" lips is an instant red flag when it comes to a natural appearance. A combination of different needles and techniques are used to modify and enhance the person's own unique lip architecture to ensure a very natural-looking appearance. Different needles will create different effects when it comes to placing Juvederm for cosmetic lip augmentation. Most needles will cause some degree of swelling and bruising, so it's best to plan ahead, as great looking lips should ideally be slowly built in, over time, and in stages to achieve the most natural appearance.

A new technique called "blunt tip cannula" is an amazing breakthrough in dermal fillers. A long and flexible needle (cannula) with a blunt tip can be inserted through one or a few small insertion points in the face. The cannula can be inserted without numbing, and can reach the entire lower face, without any bruising, swelling, or pain. This technique is new and very few providers have started using it. It's really a game changer, as anyone who has suffered days of swelling, pain and bruising can attest to. What is even more incredible is that the simple act of repeatedly inserting and filling the tissue stimulates the body's own cells, called fibroblasts to produce more collagen, naturally. (You can put aside the cow collagen now, thank goodness.)

Well-placed Juvederm can last for six months to over a year, and usually each time it is placed at subsequent visits, the filler ends up lasting longer. □

Dr. Joel Gould has been practicing in Manhattan Beach since 2001. His general and cosmetic dental office treats patients of all ages and offers a broad range of treatments. Dr. Gould owned several practices in Vancouver, Canada for 10 years before moving to the Los Angeles area, and he has trained with several Beverly Hills plastic surgeons in the art and science of Botox and Juvederm. He collaborated with Dimitri's dental studios to create the "supermodel veneer" which he uses in his instant smile makeovers. Dr. Gould recently launched his new concept called "Modern American Dentistry," a no-nonsense approach to modern dental practice. With three locations, and five dentists, he has created a dental experience that is consistently comfortable.

GYSO – Episode. 1 Jennifer Cohen

Dr. Gould: Hi, everybody out there. I am so excited to be speaking to you all. This is the premier episode of Get Your Smile On with me, Dr. Joel Gould. What I promise is it is going to be the most interesting, stimulating, and exciting internet radio show all about dentistry, but it's much bigger than that. When I decided that I was going to have a radio show the first thing I thought was, people are going to think, "Why would I want to listen to a radio show about dentistry? He's going to tell me to floss." Nothing could be further from the truth. I am not going to tell any of you to floss. I'm going to make it so that you want to.

I'm pretty excited to be here. The first thing I want to really say is who am I, and why should you care? I'm the CEO of Modern American Dentistry. We are a multi-faceted global dental brand bringing you products, exciting news, tips and tricks. I am the author of the #1 bestselling book, *The Perfect Smile*, which is released this month on Amazon. I write a column on cosmetic dentistry for Pageantry magazine that is seen in 52 countries around the world. I have treated over 250,000 patients at my practice in Canada and the US. That's a lot of people.

I'm pretty excited to be able to put everything that I know about dentistry, cosmetic dentistry, and wellness dentistry. This is my 25th year of practice in dentistry. What's important to know, and why I should be able to speak about a lot of things, is that I've had an incredible, broad range of experience, from public health dentistry, pediatrics, geriatrics, cosmetic dentistry, and I've basically reimagined, reestablished, rebuilt, multiple dental practices both in the United States and Canada. I'm here now in Southern California with my group Modern American Dentistry. We are five dentists in three locations, Northridge, Santa Monica, and Manhattan Beach, which is my flagship location. This is exactly where I'm speaking to you from, beautiful Manhattan Beach, California.

My format for my radio show is sort of interesting. I really want to make sure that I bring an exciting and interesting set of topics to discuss, and the most important part of what I'm going to talk about today is really to define what is wellness dentistry? It's interesting. Wellness dentistry is a catchall expression for what all of modern dentistry has come to be, have evolved over all these years. With 25 years' experience and experience in two countries, and all the things that I've seen and all of the interesting topics that I have covered, I really wanted to put together something that would bring dentistry into the modern age. Most people when they think about going to their dentist they've got an image of a man with a white high collared polyester coat and those funny glasses. That and pain. Let's not kid ourselves.

Dentistry has evolved in some incredible ways. If you haven't been to the dentist in a long time I hope that this will be your call to action. Dentistry is fantastic these days. It's painless. It's easy, especially at my offices. We try and make everything as accessible as possible. When you come to one of my offices, I'm not going to bother you about flossing. We're going to show you the latest tips and techniques.

So why is dentistry and wellness dentistry even important? The first and most important thing is that the mouth is an integral part of who we are. It deserves much more attention than it's getting, and what I want to do is bring attention to how to get it healthy and to keep your mouth healthy in the easiest way possible. Why is the mouth so important? Some obvious things. Your mouth is where you take in nourishment. Think of all the great meals you've had. It's how you communicate. Think of all the important people you've spoken to, and all the incredible things that you can say. It's how we reveal our outward expressions. It's how we become intimate, when you think about kissing.

If you are not confident about your smile, it can affect every aspect of who you are. People will not even want to smile. They'll cover with their hand. That's the type of thing where we start to realize just how important what your smile looks like and how you feel about it really is. Someone who's not confident about their smile will smile less, and smiling less is really just telling the general public and people that you meet that you're not that friendly. I think that nobody wants to come out of the gate saying, "I'm not that friendly." When you are happy and confident with how your teeth look, how your lips look, how your smile is, you're just going to be a happier, better, more communicative person.

Dentistry has come a long way. We're not just dealing with teeth. We're dealing with all of the important structures that are associated. Dentists study head and neck anatomy. We study with medical doctors. We really are doctors of the mouth. As a cosmetic dentist, what that means is that I look at everything. I look at someone's smile from top to bottom. I see the crow's feet around their eyes and say, "We can change that." I see the frown lines and number 11s between their eyes and know that I can use Botox in a really natural way to give you a youthful and refreshed look.

We can use something called Juvederm, which is a dermal filler, and, yes, you may have all seen episodes of whatever show where someone has their lips just too bit, that is not our goal. My goal is to enhance and refresh, and not to pervert with excess. These are things that people have on their minds. They're worried that when they have Botox they're going to look funny, or if they have their lips taken care of they're going to look weird. What I do, and what most good cosmetic and wellness dentists do, is we bring you back to the original you. If it's been a long time, and you're looking tired, we can bring your smile back to a rejuvenated look. So when I do my lip augmentations, and, yes, that is dermal filler, like Juvederm, injected into the lips, what we're going for is a restoration or an enhancement of your own natural and beautiful smile.

Those are two elements that I bring to dentistry, and when you think about the face and what you do with your jaw and your mouth, think about the muscles that you use to elevate and close your mouth. Think about clenching and grinding, the muscles that you activate when you're clenching and grinding. They're all over your head and neck. This is much more far-reaching than just looking at your teeth. I do an incredible treatment for migraines and TMJ pain where I inject Botox all down the head. It sounds terrible, but it's really not painful.

Today I really wanted to define what it is about dentistry that I want to bring to the table, and some of topics I'm going to be talking about. I am excited, because we have a fantastic guest who I'm excited is going to be my first guest on the show. We'll get to her shortly. Just to give you an idea of what kind of things I'll be discussing, and just considering that there is a link between periodontal disease or gum disease and Alzheimer 's disease. This isn't just that we think. This is something that we know. That's a game changer. If you have a very small gum infection, that infection will cause a completely out of proportion reaction in your body, causing inflammation. There are studies that prove that periodontal disease untreated will help to initiate and to make Alzheimer's disease worse.

The link between HPV, Human Papilloma Virus, and oral cancer is really shocking. In future episodes I'm going to talk about the vaccines that you can have your children be vaccinated with to avoid oral cancer. Oral cancer and HPV, Human Papilloma Virus, is one of the biggest news topics that you're going to be hearing about in the future. This isn't a sexual thing. This is a health thing. If you think about the cost involved for women to be treated with Pap smears and the cervical cancer, it's astronomical. We are now adding in oral cancer, which is increasing in everyone, not just smokers and drinkers. We know they're at risk, but now everyone's at risk. In a future show look forward to me giving you the details of what you can do to avoid oral cancer or limit your risk.

Another incredibly important healthcare topic is sleep apnea. This is one of my most fantastic, shocking, and scary topics to talk about. I'm going to discuss this with all of my listeners, and I want to bring this one out slowly, because sleep apnea, and particularly untreated, undiagnosed sleep apnea, is one of the largest public health issues that is going to affect our time. I can't wait to give you, my listeners, the jump on what you need to know to stay healthy. It's really serious stuff, and I can't wait to discuss that one.

Dr. Oz says that your silver fillings are killing you. Now is that really true? I have the answers. I can tell you the real truth about whether you should remove your fillings or not, whether they're making you sick or not, or whether that's just pure entertainment without any basis in science.

We've also got topics that include anti-aging dentistry, and I'm going to reveal some really incredible things that everyone can do to keep themselves, their face, their smile, looking young and beautiful. We're going to discuss TMJ, temporomandibular joint. Yes, you all have two of them, one on the right side and one on the left side, but everyone calls clenching and grinding TMJ. I'm going to give you the latest and most interesting information about TMJ and what you can do if you are having a problem with it. This is closely linked to migraines. We've got new great treatments that you can have at the dental office where we can treat your migraines with Botox.

The last topic that I'm really also excited to bring to you is something called the clear aligner revolution. This is something I call invisible orthodontics. Clear aligners are a system of clear plastic trays that are custom fabricated just for you that accomplish almost exactly the same thing as regular fixed metal brackets, railroad tracks. Clear aligners have revolutionized orthodontics, because the amount of people who are willing to be accepting to having a year or year and a half treatment has gone through the roof. It has increased about 75%, and this increase started pretty much exactly after the FDA approved clear aligners such as Invisalign and Clear Correct. When the FDA approved these we started to see orthodontics just about go through the roof. I'm really excited to show you what really has changed in dentistry. Something as simple as orthodontics has evolved to a whole different state.

I'll get to that topic shortly. Today my guest is going to be the incredible Jennifer Cohen, and Jennifer Cohen is a #1 bestselling author. She is a leading fitness authority, TV personality, and she appears regularly on television. She's been on The Doctors and Extra and Good Morning, America. Today I want her to be able to tell all of you about her incredible new book, *Strong is the New Skinny*. She's an incredible person. She's just had her second child, and the future of what you're going to see from her is showing how to get your baby body back into shape. Pretty fantastic. Do we have Jennifer here on the line?

Maria: No, Jennifer isn't here just yet. This is Maria DiGiovanni, and I wanted to welcome you to FoReRadio and thank you so much. I will let you know when she comes on.

Dr. Gould: Thank you, Maria. I got a bit off my clear aligners talk, because there's something more that I really want to say about it. Now, I have had a problem, and it's funny, because I'm going to take you through a personal journey. I'm not prepared to reveal exactly all the things that I have in store based on what I've been through, but what I can tell you is that I did not wear my grinding guard, my TMJ grinding guard, and I'm bad. I told all my patients to wear theirs, but I didn't wear mine. When did I remember to wear it? I woke up in the middle of the night with my teeth stuck together, in terrible pain. I woke up, sat straight up, and thought, "What the heck am I doing? Where is my grinding guard? I'm telling all my patients to wear it."

Luckily, I keep it pretty close by. I put it in. Unfortunately, what happened is I kind of destroyed my own bite, and all my teeth shifted. The biggest issue is that I had to go back into orthodontics. I went to my favorite orthodontist, Dr. Patti Panucci here in Manhattan Beach, who set me up with a set of regular old-school braces, but they were clear brackets. After the second or third week of my lips being cut to pieces, I went back to her, and I said, "Patty, cut these off."

Now we've got Jennifer on the line here. I'm going to tell you much more of the clear aligners story, because it really is revolutionary and will change people's lives. Jennifer Cohen, are you on the line?

Jennifer: I sure am, Joel.

Dr. Gould: It's so great to hear your voice. I want to let everybody know, I sort of sold you before you got on the line. I told everybody how great you are.

Jennifer: Wow. Thank you, Joel.

Dr. Gould: Well, you're great. I said your new book, *Strong is the New Skinny*, pretty fantastic stuff. I'm excited for everybody to get it, but I also let everybody know that you've just had your second baby, and what probably we're going to see from you, I'm hoping, is a book on how to lose the baby fat. You've probably already done it, haven't you?

Jennifer: I haven't done it yet, but I am planning to, and I am working on it currently. So, yes, you definitely are on the right track there.

Dr. Gould: No pressure. No pressure at all. You are probably going to be the most interesting, exciting guess that I have, and you're one of my best friends. I want to have you on the show more than once, so I hope you're going to be okay with this. What I want to do just today is—

Jennifer: With an intro like that, Joel, how can I ever say no?

Dr. Gould: You could, but you're not going to. Jennifer Cohen is a fantastic person that I met when I first moved to Los

Angeles 15 years ago. The back story here is important, because I have this radio show exclusively because Maria DiGiovanni wanted to produce it for me, and I met her through Safe Passage, which any of you who don't know is a battered women's shelter, and it's not just a place for women to go for help. It's a place that helps women get back on their feet. For myself, growing up my father was a divorce attorney back in the 70s. He was a defender of women at a time when there really weren't any. My father helps Jennifer's mother out of a terrible situation, and he helped her become more comfortable. So he's doing the type of things that Safe Passage is doing now. So for me the connection is really easy.

When I came to LA my father called me, and he said, "Joel, I want you to listen to me very carefully." Yes, that's the way my dad talks, because I'm going to quote him. He's a pretty hysterical character. He said, "I have a number for you. Her name is Jennifer Cohen, and she's very busy. She's very important, and you need to call her." I'll never forget just the way he said it, because I had this idea in my mind of this really busy, important Hollywood person, which you are, but you're also one of the most real and down to earth people that I've ever met. I told you, Jennifer. I asked you if I could say anything, and you said yes. You said I could say anything. I wanted everyone to understand that you're somebody that I have known since I came to LA 15 years ago. You have been with me through thick and thin, sickness, health, and really for better or for worse, richer or poorer. We kind of have a little bit of a history. We're not married.

Jennifer: It sounds like we are. For richer, for poorer, for sickness and in health.

Dr. Gould: We've been through a lot together, and I'm so excited for what you've done for yourself and your career, and I really wanted the opportunity to let all your fans know the other side of you. This is very different. I'm a wellness dentist, and who knows what this is? I've sort of defined it. Then people are going to find out that what I have to offer is really interesting. What I have to offer is bringing in the most incredible people on to my show, and here you are.

Jennifer: You are also an incredible dentist. Let's not forget that part.

Dr. Gould: Right. That is one portion, my shameless promotional portion. Jennifer, go for it. I'll give you 30 seconds to tell everybody how awesome I am.

Jennifer: No, you are. You're very meticulous. You're very particular, and you are a perfectionist, which of course anybody would like that when somebody's working in their mouth. I wasn't getting paid to say that. That's just the way I feel.

Dr. Gould: Right. You didn't read the notes that I gave you about what to say about me.

Jennifer: No. You didn't pass me $20 somewhere along the line. That's for sure.

Dr. Gould: Maybe one of your favorite salads at one of your favorite restaurants.

Jennifer: Maybe, if I get to be that lucky.

Dr. Gould: Tell me. I want to talk to you about multiple different topics, but because today is the first show that I'm putting on I really want you to introduce yourself, because I'm going to be calling you back here, a health, wellness, and fitness expert. I want you to say whatever you want to say about yourself to all my listeners, and I want you to talk about your new book. Go for it.

Jennifer: Really I usually have a situation where people ask me particular questions, but really I just write about anything, depending on what you're talking about. I have a column in Forbes, which is all about motivation and basically helping people be productive and live a healthier lifestyle when you're really busy, for entrepreneurs. Then I also have a column in Health magazine, which is all about fitness and ways to be fit, different fitness routines, diet, stuff like that. Then my second book is called *Strong is the New Skinny*, which is really all about taking your fitness to the next level and really changing the idea of what it is to be fit and healthy and making your goal about strength and things that are achievable versus just skinny. I think that that's kind of an old way of...

Dr. Gould: I wanted to say, I read your book, and you really couldn't have said it better, because so many people in fitness are focused on what the end result is, and I read your book, and what struck me about it is how easy the things that you talk about are to integrate into your life, because the idea that someone's going to stop what they're doing, go to the gym and spend four hours there to get fit is ridiculous. You have all these incredible tips and ways to sort of work fitness into your life.

Jennifer: Exactly. The whole philosophy is based around maximizing your effort in the minimum amount of time, and not really having to go—my first book was called *No Gym Required*, which was all about the same message, which is always the same, which is ways to integrate fitness into your life easily that works for you. You can really get just the same quality of workout being at your home as you do going to a gym, if you're doing things properly, and you can also eliminate the half an hour, 40 minutes, whatever drive time it takes to get there and all the costs that come with it.

Making small changes in your life, tweaking your lifestyle just a little bit here and there adds to big, big change. Really it's about just taking shortcuts to get to the best version of yourself and to be the healthiest version of yourself. I like the idea of people having goals like how much stronger they can be, or pushing themselves that way, versus focusing on something like being skinny. The reality is not everybody can be skinny, but everyone can be strong.

Dr. Gould: Fantastic. The reason I think that you're such an incredible guest that I want to have you back is because several of my topics have contents that really affects a lot of the things that you do and that you're into. One of the things I talk about in my anti-aging dentistry is hormone replacement, and a lot of what you do has a strong interaction with my theory and my ideas of something like HGH precursors or antecedents. That's something I'm going to talk about in another show, but that can affect everything, especially your workouts.

Jennifer: 100%. Also, as you get older, you're going to probably talk about at some point, your HGH does decline, and that affects everything in your body as well.

Dr. Gould: Yeah. Your HGH actually peaks at the age of 17, if that isn't disappointing enough to hear.

Jennifer: That is very disappointing.

Dr. Gould: Sorry. I've got some really incredible, natural, great and incredible ways that you can boost your HGH, in addition to, as you know as you stay very clear on all your material, is that exercise is really the key to boosting your immune system and your overall health. I'm really excited to bring out some of these topics that I think people may have heard of here and there and other places, but they don't really understand the details. What I want to do, what I want to bring to wellness dentistry, is I want to encapsulate all this noise that you hear out there in the world, and I want to really refine it and bring out and give back the most concise and clear easy to incorporate message, so that whatever topic we're discussing you've got a take home message. That's one of my mandates of this show is I want everybody who listens to it to walk away with something that they can incorporate into their life.

Jennifer: That's great.

Dr. Gould: This is only a half hour show, because I told all of my friends I'm going to make it as interesting and exciting as possible in a half hour, because an hour is a long time to commit to listening to a podcast.

Jennifer: So what can I give you in the next five minutes? What kind of interesting tidbit can I give you?

Dr. Gould: Let's have one tip to give our listeners that they can do right now, today or tomorrow, they can incorporate to make them just healthier and just one bit better?

Jennifer: I'll give you something super easy that anyone can do starting tonight or tomorrow. When they wake up in the morning, tomorrow when you wake up, try doing just basic 10 pushups. You can do it on your knees, or you can do it on your toes, but it's a good way to get your blood flowing starting off the day right with doing something that's for you that is going to help you get to your goal. Anyone can. It takes you 20 seconds. It takes you 30 seconds. I think anyone can find the time. If you have time to brush your teeth, you have time to do 10 pushups. Then we can move on from there.

Dr. Gould: I love it. I think that's so great, because that could really get your day going, and I know 10 pushups doesn't sound like a lot, but if you do it and you haven't been doing pushups you sure feel it right away, don't you?

Jennifer: 100%, and also it's about little wins, baby steps. I'm not going to tell somebody tomorrow to run a marathon, but if you start with something that not only is achievable but it's very easy to incorporate, because it takes such a small amount of time. You're not even leaving your bedroom by that point. It will set your day off on the right foot, and the idea would be that the next choices, the next decisions you'll make, you'll be much more cognizant to make a healthy one.

Dr. Gould: Wow. Jennifer, you are a super star. I know I read your Forbes magazine articles all the time, and there's always something really interesting and exciting to incorporate into your life, and so anybody can find Jennifer Cohen at JenniferCohen.com, just like it should be. Look her up. Her website's incredibly detailed.

Jennifer: Or at Therealjencohen.

Dr. Gould: Therealjencohen. There you go. I learned something too today.

Jennifer: Therealjencohen is Instagram, Facebook, and Twitter and all that.

Dr. Gould: Fantastic. Jennifer, I want to thank you so much for being on my show. This really means a lot to me to have, first of all, somebody who is as dynamic as you are and who's as well read, well-traveled, and an expert in your field. It really makes me feel like I'm starting off like my 10 pushups, on the right foot to getting going with my radio career.

Jennifer: You've done a great job. I'm impressed. I'm impressed. Howard Stern should be watching out for you. You're going to be nipping at his heels pretty soon.

Dr. Gould: Right? And I've got better hair than he's got. That's for sure.

Jennifer: There you go. You're on the right track right there.

Dr. Gould: Jennifer, thank you so much. I'm going to say goodbye to you. We're almost out of time, and everyone look her up. See you soon.

Jennifer: Thank you, bye.

Dr. Gould: Bye. Okay, everybody, thank you so much. If listeners want to call in to future shows we've got a number for you. It's 347-857-3670. You can find it on Facebook and all kinds of other places where anybody under the age of 21 has a hard time figuring out. I want to sign out by saying my notable line that I haven't said yet. All dentistry is cosmetic. We can't separate what looks good from what feels good. It's just impossible. So when you go to your dentist, and they say, "Is it necessary? Is it cosmetic or is this functional?" the answer really is that all dentistry is cosmetic. Our mouths are much too integrated into who we are as people for us to be able to separate something like that. That's an insurance phrase. That doesn't count in who we are. Your mouth is a giant part of who you are as a person. It's all the things that make wellness dentistry important to everybody.

I'm just about out of time. I want to thank everybody for listening, and I really promise to give you some incredible and exciting topics. Please look us up at ModernAmericanDentistry.com. You can follow us on Twitter and Facebook and all of that stuff. I can't wait to hear what some of my viewers would want to have me talk about. I'm pretty excited, and on that note I'm going to sign out. It's been great talking to you all. All dentistry is cosmetic.

GYSO – Eps. 2 Dr. Jay Sordean

Dr. Gould: That's me. Hello, and welcome back, hopefully, to some of you who are back again to Get Your Smile On with me, Dr. Joel Gould, your wellness dentist. Last week was my first show, and I really had a great time. I want to thank Maria DiGiovanni, my producer for helping me out to get on to this incredible opportunity to share wellness dentistry with the world. I'm going to just go back and say that, remember, all dentistry is cosmetic. Cosmetic because how you feel about yourself is so integrated into your smile and who you are that we just can't separate function from looking and feeling good.

Last week we had the incredible Jennifer Cohen on the show. She is a health, wellness, and fitness expert. We were talking about her new book, *Strong is the New Skinny*. It's a really great book. Just the title alone tells you that this is really somebody to watch in the health and wellness industry.

Thank you all for tuning in to what, again, I promise is going to be the most exciting half an hour internet show on dentistry. We are available now on SoundCloud under the name Dr. Joel Gould. You can look me up, and we are coming soon to iTunes.

Today my guest is going to be Dr. Jay Sordean of the Redwood Clinic in Berkeley, and he'll be on the show just a little bit later. The topic for today's show is the link between Alzheimer's disease and gum disease. I know that sounds really strange, but, again, wellness dentistry can be anything as slight as having pain, a toothache with your mouth, to as far reaching as being linked to Alzheimer's disease. Now hopefully a lot of you have seen the movie with Julianne Moore in her role as Still Alice, and that brought widespread attention to Alzheimer's disease. 5.2 million Americans currently have Alzheimer's disease, and probably everyone listening has somebody in their life that has been touched by this disease or knows somebody who's being affected by it today.

What's really interesting about this disease is, as a dentist, I have a unique position to be seeing people every six months over many years, and it's really sad for me when I see one of my formerly fantastic, great, really vital patients just slowly start to deteriorate. At a certain point the patients themselves are really not feeling pain. They're really not sure about a lot, but it's the loved ones that have to help and carry on, and it can be really tough. We get a lot of people coming in to continue their dental care, bringing in their loved ones who are affected by this disease, and I know it affects so many people. As an aging population in America, by the year 2050 the number of people with Alzheimer's disease will triple, and that's due to the giant amount of people in the baby boom generation.

Today's topic, I promised that I wouldn't use this as an opportunity to bug you about flossing, because when you come to a dental office that's probably one of the first things that you think we're going to do, and that is going to be to say, "You're not flossing enough." One of the things that I really want to do with this show is not tell you about anything. I really want everybody to learn something from either the guests that we have on or some of the statistics that I'm going to speak about or some of the ideas and information that I'm going to bring forward, because I want everybody who's listening to understand dentistry and health the way I understand.

One of my biggest topics that we're going to be talking about is one that is really interesting that people have an issue with this already. It's called sleep apnea. I really want to rename that to sleep disorders. Apnea is a weird word, and a lot of people have heard of it, and they're just not interested. They know that they don't have, or they believe they don't have it, and people who know what sleep apnea is they picture a giant gas mask that's blowing air down their throat.

The people of you who don't know what sleep apnea is, it's different than insomnia, although 80% of insomniacs have sleep apnea. What it is is an obstruction of your airway. There's a lot to this whole phenomenon, and it's an incredible, complex, intriguing, terrifying issue that I'm going to be bringing forward to my show little by little. It's one of the biggest healthcare issues facing our time, and I'm here to be at the forefront of helping to identify what is sleep apnea, what sleep disorders are, and at the forefront of treating them.

Why would a dentist be treating a sleep disorder? Many, many reasons. Just briefly, the dentists that are out there we see people's airways. We look at their teeth, and we see their tongues and their tonsils. Sure, when you go to the doctor they'll use that tongue depressor and look down your throat, but we have you lying back. We can see it all. We are uniquely positioned to be able to see the early warning signs of sleep apnea. I don't want to go too far into this, but sleep apnea is considered a period of time where you actually stop breathing, and your body goes into alarm mode, and it wakes you up. One of the conditions that sleep apnea makes worse is Alzheimer's disease.

We will get back to sleep apnea. We're going to discuss it quite a bit. We are starting in my office a clinical trial, and I have a very unique link to this disease, sleep apnea, as I was actually diagnosed with it. It was a complete shock to me. I was in total denial. I had been to many continuing education seminars where I learned about how to treat people with sleep apnea. In fact, we've been doing it for many years here. The issue is that I think a lot of people and a lot of dentists didn't really understand or don't really understand how complex this is, and pretty much only through me really having this has sort of enabled me to have a completely different focus and view on it.

I'm getting into some of the incredible science that is going to change people's ideas of what sleep apnea is into more of what sleep disorders are, and we can hopefully bring to light that there are a lot of other solutions besides the C-pap machine, which is the big gas mask that you see, but we can do something called a mandibular advancement device. The acronym is MAD, just like Modern America Dentistry, MAD. I'm really mad for MADs because I am looking forward to getting probably the first good night's sleep I've ever had in my entire life. I don't have my MAD or my dental device yet, but it's on its way.

Today we're discussing Alzheimer's disease, and we have our guest today is Dr. Jay Sordean, and I'm going to bring him on in a second. He is a really incredible guy. He is an LAC, Licensed Acupuncturist. He's an OMD, Oriental Medicine Doctor. He's a CTN, Certified Traditional Naturopath. He's a QME, a Qualified Medical Evaluator, and just to throw a few more letters at you, he's been seen on CBS, NBC, ABC, and FOX, however you want to say it.

He has a book that we're going to get him to talk about. He and I have known each other for a while. We've discussed the complications of Alzheimer's disease and how it's linked to oral health, and I would like to bring him on. Dr. Jay, are you there?

Dr. Jay: Hi, Joel. It's great to be on the air tonight with you.

Dr. Gould: Thank you very much. We didn't get a lot of a chance to talk about this in advance, and I'm not sure how much you know about this show, but we are not yet on iTunes, but hopefully by the end of next week we'll be listed. Your people who want to hear what you have to say can find us on SoundCloud under Dr. Joel Gould. Dr. Jay, I've seen you on TV, and you're a compelling speaker. I think you're entertaining. I think you're exciting. Tell us about your new book.

Dr. Jay: I actually have two books. One is called *Super Brain, Maximize Your Brain Health for a Better Life,* and that's a bit more about enhancing the brain, as well as trying to avoid Alzheimer's and dementia. The other is called *Outsmarting the Dementia Epidemic,* because I feel very strongly that this 1 in 8 Americans epidemic of Alzheimer's is something that needs to be addressed, just as diabetes and obesity need to be addressed as well.

Dr. Gould: That's your more recent book.

Dr. Jay: That's correct. Some of the factors, when we jump right into talking about Alzheimer's, some of the factors related to Alzheimer's and brain degeneration include a decreased oxygen getting to the brain, a lack of REM sleep, which prevents restorative sleep and memory processing, and obesity and blood sugar conditions. These all are factors that science and research have shown, as well as clinical studies have shown, have an influence on causing brain degeneration and impact Alzheimer's. Now one of the interesting things is some of the factors and symptoms in Alzheimer's dementia patients include the sundowner phenomenon of waking and not being able to sleep. So there's a certain parallel with sleep apnea in a number of these different issues having to do with, perhaps you already stated that sleep apnea tends to reduce the oxygenation to the brain, and one of theories is that a decrease in the steady flow of oxygen to the brain is one of the negative effects that sleep apnea has on a person's health.

Dr. Gould: Sure. I didn't get into, sleep apnea is such a broad subject. What I really have been trying to do is just break it in slowly. What's so interesting is that Alzheimer's is definitely linked to sleep apnea. The two are really parallel in a lot of ways. I want to get to this, but right now we actually have just a short break for one of our commercials, and we're going to take a break for one second. Hang in there, and we'll get right back to you.

Okay. Sorry about that, Jay. This is my second show, and introducing a commercial break is something that's new to me. Thanks for bearing with me. I did not want to lose the momentum of what we're talking about, but I want to just change gears real quick. I just want to say that we had discussed this issue of Alzheimer's disease and dental health. What's interesting is that since you and I spoke in detail the research that I did showed that this isn't just any kind of suggestion. There's a conclusive and interesting link between periodontal disease and Alzheimer's that is actually separate from the whole sleep apnea and decreased oxygen issue. Is that correct?

Dr. Jay: It is certainly the research that I have done. I know that in my TV segments I mentioned the importance of dental hygiene, reducing inflammation and bacterial infection, because that has a global effect. It can also have a localized effect on the sinuses, and those can eventually cause what we call leaky brain syndrome.

Dr. Gould: Yikes.

Dr. Jay: Which is damage to the filtration system that protects the brain. When that happens all kinds of very degenerative processes occur in the brain, a lot of inflammation. Dealing with the dental hygiene is so crucial in this whole picture, and it's not being looked at by most physicians.

Dr. Gould: Right. I totally agree with you, and I promised that this show would be as exciting as possible. I didn't want to say things, but this is actually really on point, is that everybody out there if you're not seeing a dentist regularly go see one. If you're near me, come to one of my three offices. We do all manner of periodontal care, deep cleanings, everything that you need at the right frequency. Some people need more cleaning. Some people need less. It depends on who you are, but it's very important.

Even leaving a wisdom tooth that's halfway into your mouth can cause a chronic periodontal infection, and what the studies showed that I was most shocked at is that this small periodontal infection that you have in your mouth will trigger a completely out of size response from your immune system. Your immune system kind of goes crazy. A small periodontal infection isn't that big. It's not that big of a deal. It won't affect your life, but it really gets the immune system going, which really has to do with back to the topics of Alzheimer's, sleep apnea, and oxygen deprivation.

Dr. Jay: So true. One of the things that I was talking to someone recently, and her partner worked at Memorial Sloan Kettering, and he is a dentist. The reason why the whole dental component is in that facility is because cancer patients, when their immune system gets lowered, they have some of the worst dental problems, and that will eventually be one of the major causes of death. So this, again, points out the real key requirement that people get their teeth looked at, that they have regular dental care as a part of overall health, but also even for things such as cancer. I know we aren't talking about that here, but it is a key factor in taking care of people who have cancer and advanced cancer.

Dr. Gould: Thank you for making my dental claims for me. I think that's great. I appreciate it. What I want to do right now, you're such an interesting guy, and you do so many things, basically we said if you didn't need one more reason to floss, there it is. If you don't floss, you can get Alzheimer's disease. Not to scare you, but physical health, dental health, and overall well-being is really critical to your overall health.

What I wanted to do, Jay, is I want to just talk about some of the things that people don't know maybe about you, probably don't know. I know you do a lot of work with acupuncture. What is your most common treatment that you do for acupuncture? Tell us a little about that.

Dr. Jay: Acupuncture historically in the United States has primarily focused on pain control, because of the trips that President Nixon did to China, and James Reston who was a reporter had observed people having surgery using acupuncture. So a lot of people come to my office related to pain problems. It could be headaches. It could be digestive issues, even tooth pain. Of course, they have to get the dentist to make sure that the underlying cause is being addressed as well, but there are a lot of different points and areas in the teeth that correspond to different organs in the body, and so treating with acupuncture can help the teeth as well be healthy and to help the dental care be more effective.

Dr. Gould: Okay. Sorry, go on.

Dr. Jay: I also work with people who—

Dr. Gould: Hello?

Dr. Jay: Yeah.

Dr. Gould: Are we there? Okay. Sorry, you cut out there for a second. Go on.

Dr. Jay: Individuals who need to lose weight is an important thing. One of the things that I work with, because it has to do with overall metabolism, overall function of the body, and if blood sugar is out of balance that can create all kinds of havoc. If one looks on the internet and other places under sleep apnea, what also is commonly stated is that obesity is a major cause of sleep apnea and that problem, because of the swelling and all the extra weight that occurs, the extra tissue structure that occurs, it's difficult to breathe when you're asleep. So actually treating obesity as one aspect is very important in dealing with sleep apnea, but it's a key component in dealing with Alzheimer's, because of blood sugar issues going up and down causing inflammation, and then that can involve the brain as well and cause brain degeneration.

Dr. Gould: Right. Okay. Again, sleep apnea is such a big topic, and I really want to roll it out slowly that people can get how far this reaches into our current medical system, but interestingly enough, not only is sleep apnea made worse or caused by obesity, but the reverse is true as well. People who have sleep apnea will become obese, because their hormones are just completely messed up, and so the hormonal paths that signal to the brain to be satisfied or to be hungry get completely messed up.

               We'll go into that at a later show, because there's an incredible link between obesity, sleep apnea, and general hormones. So being fit and being healthy is completely related to that. We'll save that. Unfortunately the sleep apnea conversation just sneaks in everywhere, because it's just linked to so many different things. Tell me, for your patients that you do treat with acupuncture, is it a long session? Do you see them for 10 minutes? How does it go?

Dr. Jay: Initially, in order to get a great overview of all the health issues that are going on with an individual, because there could be emotional issues, there could be things that are going on in their relationships that are influencing their overall health. I do a comprehensive evaluation, and often that will be an hour, hour and a half, long, depending on what's going on. If they're coming in with pain problems I have to do a proper orthopedic evaluation. I have to do range of motion, testing out muscle strength, etc. So for most people the first visit is anywhere from a half hour to an hour and a half, so I can get a complete picture of what's going on.

Many people will come in after having seen a lot of other physicians, and they may have a huge stack of different laboratory tests or x-rays, and often times we have to do additional testing that has not been done, in order to find out what is going on functionally with them. It could have to do with hair mineral analysis. It may have to do with special blood tests, or it could have to do with the whole digestive system and seeing how well that is working, and whether there is an imbalance of the bacteria in the intestinal track that is causing all kinds of other problems and weakening their immune system, for example. So that's the first visit.

Dr. Gould: Okay. I know you touched on about a million different topics that are of interest.

Dr. Jay: I did.

Dr. Gould: It's tough to get it all in, but so tell me about your treatment. As dentists, someone comes in, and we do our set of x-rays, just like you're talking about. We do a history, and we come up with something called a treatment plan. It varies from person to person. A lot of people don't need any work, and a lot of people need to have their mouths completely redone. So what we do is make up a treatment plan. We phase it. We're say we're going to do this, this, or this. Does that type of thing work the same with acupuncture? Do you have to have a repeated treatment? What would your first acupuncture visit be once you decided that that's going to be a proper treatment modality?

Dr. Jay: Exactly. Once I determine that it's a possibility, some people have come in they've already had acupuncture, so we know that it has some beneficial affects to them. Not everyone is a perfect candidate for acupuncture, but many people actually do find that acupuncture is helpful for them, for a variety of reasons. So typically if I haven't seen someone before, in order to see if they're a fast or slow responder I would need to at least six visits, and then by then I would know whether they were going to respond quickly or more slowly, or they don't respond at all to the acupuncture I do.

Then from there, depending on how severe the problem is, how impacted it is in their system, it could take 12 visits. It could take 24 visits. There are individuals I have seen who came in, I've practiced more than 33 years, and so I think maybe 28 years ago there's a person that I had been seeing that long, and they were able to avoid back surgery. Still haven't had to have back surgery, and they will come in occasionally for tune ups. They say, "I felt a little twitch." So they come in.

Dr. Gould: That's really interesting. How long have you been doing the acupuncture for? You've been doing it for 33 years?

Dr. Jay: For 33 years.

Dr. Gould: Wow. Okay. Usually this where I make a comment like I've got underwear older than 33 years, but I'm not wearing them tonight.

Dr. Jay: You aren't wearing those. Those are up on the wall somewhere in a museum.

Dr. Gould: There you go. Exactly. Now, as a naturopathic doctor, so obviously we know that you do acupuncture, what other types of things do you think that people listening who don't what you do would be surprised to find that you do, or that you do well, or that you love to do, or that's unusual or beneficial?

Dr. Jay: As a naturopath as well as an acupuncturist, I work with homeopathic remedies. I work with herbs, and they can be Chinese herbal formulas or Western style, depending on what's necessary. There are nutraceuticals that I use that are based on biological medicine.

Dr. Gould: Hold on one second. What's a nutraceutical?

Dr. Jay: A nutraceutical is a nutrient that has been specifically, either an extract or a formulation, that is based on natural medicine. It has exacting, it's like we know the percentage of the active ingredients in it.

Dr. Gould: Okay. Got it. So basically you do sort of more scientific based as well as more Eastern medicine based type of treatment then?

Dr. Jay: That's exactly right. I also do something called neurologic release center technique, which is working with the meninges, and that is something I've been doing in addition to the acupuncture over the last five years. I decided to do that because I saw some really miraculous changes that occurred when people's meninges, which are like three layers of plastic wrap—

Dr. Gould: Hold on. I'm going to interrupt you just so that everybody, I'm pretty sure that everybody listening doesn't necessarily know what the meninges are. So it sounds like maybe a Saturday morning cartoon.

Dr. Jay: That's right.

Dr. Gould: This is the material that lines people's brains. Is that correct? Did I say it right?

Dr. Jay: That's right. It's like three layers of Saran Wrap, or plastic wrap, that surrounds the brain, every little crevice in the brain, as well as all the nerves coming off of the spinal cord and off of the brain stem. It's sort of like having three wet suits on a person, if you've ever been out surfing or something. It's like three wet suits. So if they get twisted or torqued, then it can affect the blood flow going to the brain, the oxygen going to the brain, and the cerebrospinal fluid which circulates through the spine and the brain in order to nourish it and to have the immunological factors necessary to protect it.

Dr. Gould: Wow. So what kind of treatment do you do for that?

Dr. Jay: That is a manual treatment where we actually apply pressure in various parts of the neck in order to release the twisted or torqued meninges. It sounds radical, but it's subtle, and yet I have seen these really amazing changes. People who had hip pain for 20 years after like a three week series of treatments they're hip pain, actually right after the first visit they go, I can't believe I don't have any hip pain after 20 years. It's like, I'm going, just adjusting. I often go, is this really working that well? I mean, it's like, I can't believe it.

Dr. Gould: I want to interrupt you there, because I've been taking some training in trigger points. I'm like an old-school scientist, so if anyone says anything that's sort of out of line with what I think science is I get all upset. There's a lot of stuff, and naturopathics are sure in that world, but there's a lot of stuff that really became clear to me when I actually did trigger point injections, and we did this head and neck area for people who were having chronic pain. Really shocking to see how an injection of lidocaine or Botox, or even just the actual using the needle, called dry needling, can relieve, and you can feel something so far away from the actual source that it really kind of blew my mind. I really have become much more open to the whole idea that the body is such a weird interconnected place.

Dr. Jay, I'm sorry to cut you off. We're nearing the end of our show. You've got so many incredible things to talk about. I would love you have you on my show again, and I want to really thank you for your time, and I look forward to seeing you soon.

Dr. Jay: My great pleasure. Thanks for inviting me.

Dr. Gould: It was fun. Thank you.

Dr. Jay: Thanks a lot.

Dr. Gould: Okay. Everybody, today we're just about done for the day. I hope I didn't bug you to floss too much, but that is my job. I want to thank ForeRadio for sponsoring my show, and Living Royal Productions, and I would ask you all to tune in next week, 7:00PM. Hopefully by then we'll be up on iTunes. Remember, all dentistry is cosmetic. It was great talking to you tonight. We'll see you soon.

GYSO – Eps. 3
Dr. Paul Knittel Emergency Medicine

Dr. Gould: All right, everybody, welcome to tonight's show. We are in beautiful Manhattan Beach, California, and I am at my flagship location of Modern American Dentistry. Welcome to Get Your Smile on, the most exciting half hour internet radio show in existence, because I say so at this point in time, and I don't have a lot of competition. I'm excited to be speaking to everybody again. We're discussing wellness dentistry. What is wellness dentistry? Let's think of it this way. The eyes are the window to the soul. The mouth is the gateway to the entire body. We take in nourishment through our mouths. We communicate. We are able to do so many things. This is the portal to the entire body. We see what goes on in the mouth affects the entire body. We can see your airway and all kinds of interesting things.

Last week we had a really interesting show. We had Dr. Jay Sordean on, and we talked about the conclusive link between Alzheimer's disease and periodontal disease. Remember, if you didn't need one more reason to floss, there it is. The link is conclusive. So let's talk prevention, and let's talk about coming into my office, one of my offices, or your local dental office to make sure that you're staying healthy by having your teeth cleaned preventatively. Periodontal infections are minor, but they can cause a major overreaction in your immune system.

Today's topic is emergency, emergency 9-1-1, emergency dentistry, emergency medicine, and our guest for today is the emergency doctor, Dr. Paul Knittel of Dr. Paul's Emergency Care. We're going to have him on a little later in the show. I wanted to talk today about emergencies. What is classified as an emergency? What in dentistry is an emergency? Is it a filling that fell out? Is that an emergency? To some people it is, because if you can't chew, and you're in pain, then that's an emergency.

What I want to talk about today are some of the more common emergencies that are really serious. I want to divide them into two categories. One of them is uncontrollable, and the other is controllable. When I say controllable, what I mean is when it comes to the mouth, and the health of the gums and the health of the teeth, the issues that we have are when decay, and decay is an actual bacterial infection of tooth structure. When decay starts it's painless. So when someone comes to my office, and I say to them, "Mrs. Jones you've got a cavity on tooth #30." The answer for her is, "It's not hurting at all, so I'm fine. Why should I do anything about it?"

Of course, the answer really is that if we can treat teeth preventively, if we can keep them clean, brush and floss them, prevent decay from starting, then we don't have to worry about decay, but once decay starts, if we treat it quickly with a filling we can prevent further, more serious disruption of your tooth's health, and as that decay moves closer and closer to the nerve it starts to actually infect the nerve. So the bacteria that are inside the cavity start to travel down the little tiny dentinal tubules, and those are little tubes that are filled with fluid that your tooth is made up of. On the outside you have the hard enamel. On the inside you have the softer dentin. Once bacteria get into your tooth they can travel all the way down into the nerve or the pulp.

I don't want this to sound terrible or painful, but it's really important that everybody should know that an emergency would be a toothache. So with regards to prevention, if you can see a dentist, your dentist or me, and we can x-ray your teeth and we can find out what's going on, we can see decay at a really early stage. What we can do is we can do an easy inexpensive preventive treatment. If we put a small filling into a tooth we can preserve the life of that tooth. If the decay gets bigger, now we've got a much bigger filling. There's much less tooth structure, and a life of eating ice cream and hot coffee, expansion and contraction, we put our teeth through a heck of a lot. So we want to make sure we keep them as pristine as possible.

Now an emergency happens when somebody has a cavity they don't know they have. Maybe they haven't been to the dentist, or maybe they haven't been able to get dental care. So now they have extreme pain. What does that pain mean? Extreme dental pain is almost always caused by the nerve dying, and it can be very painful. Before a nerve dies it will give you some sensitivity sometimes, but most often a tooth will just all of a sudden start to be very painful. That's an emergency. That's when you call your dental office. You do not go to the emergency room.

When a tooth that needs a root canal gets really badly infected, and what that means is the infection inside the tooth has now spread to the bone, that causes an abscess. An abscess can be formed anywhere in your body where you have a bacterial infection. An abscess near a tooth is situated near the bone, where the tooth is being held, and that can be very painful. We see swelling. When swelling gets to be extreme you need to go to the emergency room. What I mean is when the swelling gets so bad it could actually close your airway. Being preventive in your care and taking care of your teeth technically could save your life.

Most infections do not cause you to have to run to the emergency room. I do want to talk about a more dangerous infection that people don't know about. It's very unusual, but when you get an infection in any of your front six teeth, those teeth drain into a different area, and an infection in those teeth can actually cause something called a cavernous sinus thrombosis. That is really bad, and that can cause death, and it's very serious. So any type of swelling or infection related to teeth you should go to your dentist right away. If it's in the front area, it's much more serious. You may want to consider, if there's no dental office open and you're nervous, you could go to the emergency room. We are going to be talking to our emergency room doctor shortly.

Now I want to talk about the other type of dental emergency, and that's trauma. Trauma is when you're at a baseball game and a fly ball comes and hits you in the face and fractures your jaw, breaks your tooth, or knocks a tooth out. We call that an avulsed tooth. I know they're all kinds of talk about what to do when a tooth gets knocked out. I'm going to tell you the secrets right now. This is most common with kids at baseball games. They'll get a tooth knocked out. You definitely want to put the tooth directly back in the kid's mouth. It depends how old they are. If it's not a permanent tooth, it's a baby tooth, then we don't worry about it.

If it's an adult tooth, so from the age of 6, 7, 8. I'd say 8 on. If you can, you can put the tooth back into the child's mouth. The saliva and that environment, even with blood, is much healthier than anything else you can do with that tooth. This tooth can be reimplanted. It can be successfully put back into the jaw and can serve for many years as a normal and natural tooth. It's really kind of unique and unusual that part of your body can come, and you can put it back in. The second best thing that you can do with a tooth is put it in some milk, a cup of milk, doesn't really matter. The third best thing would be water, clean, safe water. Get to a dentist immediately. That's when you call your dentist. If you go to an emergency room they're really not equipped to put a tooth back in. Call your local dentist. They should have an emergency number, and this is something that's very common. Most dentists deal with this all the time.

What's another type of trauma that would be an emergency? That would be a fracture of a tooth, and that can happen by biting on an olive pit or a stone. It can also happen if you are clenching and grinding too much. You can actually fracture your tooth. When a tooth fractures the pain can be extreme, and sometimes the tooth needs to be extracted. Sometimes we can do a root canal, and we can salvage the tooth, and sometimes we actually have to take the tooth completely out.

Most of the dental issues that are traumatic and serious we're going to go through two stages. The first stage is where someone's had trauma. You got hit in the face with a baseball. We're really concerned about your teeth, but we're more concerned about putting stitches in your face, and we're more concerned about the swelling and the pain that you're having. So if you don't have a tooth in your hand, but you've been hit in the face, you want to go seek emergency medical care first. Go to your emergency room first. Call your dentist second. Most of the dental work that dentists do with regards to trauma is really easily fixed within a day, two days, three days, and even five days. Totally fine.

I just want to recap here that emergencies happen in dentistry and in medicine, and they're pretty much related. When you have a very serious tooth infection we can definitely want to decide whether you have to go to the hospital or whether you're just going to go to your dentist. Common sense always rules.

I want to tell you a couple funny stories. If I get a phone call, and this is my favorite phone call, and I don't mind because I'm here to help my patients out. My favorite phone call is a phone call that I get on Friday at about 6:30PM when the office is closed, and that phone call is from somebody who's having a tooth problem, and it's always the same thing. I love it, because they leave a message and say, "Hi, Dr. Gould, I'm sorry to bother you, but I'm having an emergency. Remember that tooth that you told me I should get a crown on last year, well it broke four months ago, and about a week ago it started to hurt. Right now it really hurts."

It makes me laugh, because I bug people all the time, because I'm the only person that's going to bug my patients about their teeth, really. As dentists and dental professionals we see what's going on in your mouth, and if you don't take our recommendations that's fine, but the reality is prevention and what we recommend at dental offices is going to save you hours and a lot of money.

I'm just going to shift topics for a couple of seconds. We talked about last time as well sleep apnea and sleep disorders. I shared with everybody that I was diagnosed with a moderate to severe case of obstructive sleep apnea, and I've said this before. It's such a big topic, I want to talk about it little by little, and part of what I want to talk about today are the major emergency complications that happen with this type of thing, with sleep apnea.

What are the most urgent issues that happen with it? The two most major concerns that we have are heart attack and stroke. 90% of all heart attacks and strokes that happen at night are caused by sleep apnea, either undiagnosed or untreated sleep apnea. What does that mean? Sleep apnea is an obstruction of your airway, and when your airway is obstructed when you sleep your body actually stops breathing. You're paralyzed. To be able to wake yourself back up is very disruptive to your sleep. It's also very damaging on your body.

I want to now introduce me guest today, Dr. Paul Knittel of Dr. Paul's Emergency Care. He has over 14 years in the industry of emergency medicine. He's board certified in emergency medicine, and he has been working in Southern California's hospitals for over 14 years. Today I want to welcome Dr. Paul. Dr. Paul, how are you doing?

Dr. Paul: I'm doing well. Thank you.

Dr. Gould: I'm very happy to have you on the show. Before I let you talk, I just want to tell my listeners about what I've seen with what you're doing, and I know everyone's been to an emergency room and a primary center or emergency care. There's so many bad experiences. Just in what you do, just the general attitude is really spectacular, and I feel like you bring something to medicine in the same way that I feel like I bring something to dentistry, a warm environment where I'm interested and concerned, and every single person who walks through the door, they're a person. They're not a Mrs. Jones or a number. They're a real person. I just want to tell everybody out there that your operation has got the greatest energy, and it just looks and feels nothing like a horrible emergency room. Why don't you tell us about your current business here in South Bay?

Dr. Paul: I absolutely will. You kind of hit it right on the head. That's exactly what we were trying to accomplish is what you said. I basically was trying to take the ER out of emergency medicine and trying to bring emergency quality care to a community setting where we could probably see and treat approximately let's say 75-80% of things that I would have typically seen in the emergency room.

Dr. Gould: That sounds ridiculous. I can't believe that anybody could think—wait, sorry, hold on. What a fantastic idea. Sorry to interrupt. You go on. One of the things that you and I have talked about is that I'm Canadian, and I have experience in the Canadian healthcare system, and no system is perfect, let me tell you, but coming to the US was really a very different experience for me, because it's very different than Canada. So go ahead and tell us a little more about your business.

Dr. Paul: It's called Dr. Paul's Immediate Care, and we're located on Artesia Boulevard, conveniently located, basically at the corner of all four of the South Bay beach cities, Redondo, Hermosa, and Manhattan Beach. Our acronym is DPIC, Dr. Paul's Immediate Care, but we like to think it stands for Delivering Patients Incredible Care. Again, back to what we were talking about before.

Dr. Gould: I love it. I just want to help all of our listeners understand, because this is a global podcast. The South Bay is the area in Los Angeles, and it is the area that is south of LAX, Los Angeles airport, and it's mostly known as the beach communities of Manhattan Beach, Hermosa Beach, Redondo Beach, and these are places people have heard of, but this is where this show is coming to you from, and this is where your business is from. I just want to clarify that to everybody. I wanted to ask you, what made you get into emergency medicine?

Dr. Paul: Emergency medicine. I wanted to be a physician and go to medical school from a time before I can even remember, and as I went through my medical training and went through my rotations and explored all the different options of specialties I found that I actually really enjoyed almost all the specialties, and I found that emergency medicine would allow me to treat the widest range of patients with the widest range of problems.

Dr. Gould: That's really interesting, because as a general dentist that's sort of, a lot of dentists specialize, but you get to see everything as a general dentist. I guess I didn't think of the perspective that you'd be thinking like that. I find that really interesting. Was there one aspect? Is there a level of excitement that you like about? Is it the excitement that new things will come in through the door as well?

Dr. Paul: Definitely. It's definitely the fast paced nature of emergency medicine too that I've enjoyed. What I've really enjoyed is being able to treat people at their most critical time when I can provide them the most positive and immediate impact on their lives and their health. That's just proved to be very rewarding, and I'm excited to continue that here now in my own practice and practice in my own way that I would like, in a situation where how I want it to be run and with people that I know are good and trustworthy.

Dr. Gould: That's great. Also, I know that you guys have some different hours than the average medical practice. I know how hard it is for me to get to any medical facility, because I'm booked with patients all day. So you've got some different hours. What are you usually offering for patients?

Dr. Paul: We do. We are open Monday through Friday. We open at 8:00 in the morning, and we see patients up until about 7:00 at night. We'll take our last patient at 7:00, and we'll take as long as we need to to finish seeing you once you check in. So we provide some afterhours so it's easier for some of the working parents and people that need to get in here after work. Then we have weekend hours.

Dr. Gould: You do. Okay. I was a little nervous. You do have some weekend hours.

Dr. Paul: We do. Our weekend hours we're here from about 9:00 to 5:00PM. Again, trying to be available for the weekend accidents and illnesses.

Dr. Gould: Right. Tell me about it. We're going to go onto a short commercial break here to recognize our sponsors who are helping us to have this show. We're going to take a quick break, and we'll be right back. So hang on.

We're back. Thank you very much. Dr. Paul, we still have you on the line?

Dr. Paul: I am here.

Dr. Gould: Great. I shared with the listeners my funny story of that phone call I always get on Friday after the office is closed. This is your opportunity to tell everyone listening. What is it that you see coming into the emergency room consistently that kind of drives you crazy, that if you could tell one thing to everybody out there, this is what I want to see different or I want to point out? What would you tell people? What is it out there that you'd like to change?

Dr. Paul: That's a great question. I would say probably with overwhelming enthusiasm that people just need to stay healthy. How do you stay healthy? One of the best ways to do that is to get to sleep at a consistent time and get a specific amount of sleep every night.

Dr. Gould: Okay.

Dr. Paul: Here's the down side to emergency medicine, so this kind of funny that I'm promoting emergency medicine, but as an emergency medicine physician this became an actual personal issue for me, as we work in the ER crazy hours. So you're working overnight, graveyard shifts. You're working swing shifts late into the night. You're working extremely early hours, so starting at 6:00AM. So sleep is all over the board, and when you're sleeping irregularly and not at consistent times and consistent hours your body starts to feel that. I personally started to deal with issues of weight gain and insulin resistance, developing some early stages of diabetes. I can, like I said, with overwhelming confidence say get sleep. Get sleep.

Dr. Gould: You are my doctor, and we talked about this on the previous show that I was shockingly surprised that I have sleep apnea. The name of my new book is *Not Me, I Don't Have It*, because that's what people say. Everyone's really in denial. Why it's such a compelling topic, and I've shared this with my guests, is that sleep apnea or sleep disorders of some kind they cut across the board. They impact every health issue. They make every situation technically a lot worse. We're going to talk in future shows, because this is such a broad topic, and it's so important, that I want to really divide it up into different areas so that people can comprehend. I can say, blah, blah, blah sleep apnea all day long, and it makes most people want to run and leave the room, but the reality is that sleep disorders are affecting our society in so many different ways.

Part of the message that I have on this show, and that I've talked about, is the message of prevention. Prevention saves pain. It saves money. It saves aggravation. I asked you, when we started talking about sleep apnea, I asked you a question. I said, "What percentage of people who end coming into the ER with a heart attack or stroke are most likely have sleep apnea, either undiagnosed or untreated?" What'd you say?

Dr. Paul: You did, and I didn't give you a number, but I would say very high. It was a very high percentage, maybe even all of them. Whatever that number is it's going to be a very impressive stat and number.

Dr. Gould: Right. What I wanted to sort of focus on today is, because you are an emergency room doctor and you've seen this, aside from the gunshot wounds, which is probably very interesting, the main issues that people have are heart attack and stroke. I know that I discussed a lack of oxygen damages the blood cells, but maybe you want to give us the elevator pitch of heart attack and stroke. What's happening? What's a quick definition of those, and why would they be even affected by sleep?

Dr. Paul: Absolutely. When we talk about heart attacks, called Myocardial Infarctions. We talk about strokes, which are Intracerebral Infarctions. These are a decrease, sudden decrease, in blood flow to the heart and to the brain, with each respective disease. If you are already, not predisposed but you're already likely to have one of those acute issues, if you add sleep apnea on top of that, now you're elevating that risk of decreasing blood flow and therefore oxygen supply to your heart muscle and to your brain. It's just kind of compounding these issues.

Dr. Gould: For example, when someone has high blood pressure, why do people have high blood pressure? What are the most common causes?

Dr. Paul: Common causes of high blood pressure are obesity.

Dr. Gould: Right. Everyone knows that one.

Dr. Paul: Right, we know that one. We know diabetes has some to do with it.

Dr. Gould: We know genetic components as well.

Dr. Paul: There's genetic components, and renal disease, so kidney disease will also cause hypertension.

Dr. Gould: So what we know is that so many people who have high blood pressure are being prescribed medications, and we don't know if they've even been screened for sleep apnea or sleep disorders. So one of the mandates that I have, I've been treating sleep apnea for a while here in the office with my Mandibular Advancement Device here. I just didn't have a compelling story, and now that it's me I really do. I really want to bring to light all these important things, and I want to make sure that our listeners have an idea that this is something that can affect every single person, and it's not just whether you have it. If you're a provider for your family, and you have sleep apnea and it's either undiagnosed or untreated, you stand the risk for dying of a heart attack or stroke.

When people do come into the emergency room, is it even in the discussion? This is something that's been known for a while, but has to come to the forefront. What do you see in your situation with regards to discussion? Is this an underlying factor in what you're seeing?

Dr. Paul: I believe it's an underlying factor, and the problem is I think it's been a widely ignored diagnosis or cause or issue to these problems. I think it's something that we need to quickly turn around and start having this discussion as far as sleep apnea, as far as just talking about it, talking about getting diagnosis for it and getting treatment for it.

Dr. Gould: What's your experience been with even discussing it? Just recently, as I bring this up, I see a variety of reactions. The majority are, not me, I don't have it. I don't snore. I sleep great. These are things that I would have said, or did say. What's your experience with even discussing this with people?

Dr. Paul: I would agree. I think most people, unless you fit the classic disposition for having sleep apnea. If you're discussing it with somebody who may not think it's even a possibility that they have it, yeah, I think they're very resistant to believing that that's an issue that they might have.

Dr. Gould: For me I had the image of the heavier guy with the big neck, heavy snorer, and I thought that doesn't fit me. I think what my conversation with you that we had, and why I think this is such a huge issue, is that this is not on people's radar, and the perception of it is really not good. I want to change it. I want to call it sleep disorders, because as we'll discuss later on, there's so many different types of sleep apnea, and some of them are commonly found in women who are petite, and that's a whole different discussion. It's actually a really interesting one, because it has more to do with your REM sleep, your deep sleep, because your body has to be paralyzed. I really definitely want to bring you back and break this topic down. I know that you have a lot of important things that we can help get the public more aware.

I want to start to close the show here. We're getting to the end of our half hour. Any parting advice that you want to give to everybody out there who's coming to your emergency room? Get a good night's sleep.

Dr. Paul: Get that good night's sleep. Eat a healthy diet. Get your exercise in, so you can get that good night's sleep. I think that's a great start as far as maintaining overall general good health.

Dr. Gould: Great. It's just reinforcement of the prevention really is everything. Dr. Paul, I want to thank you so much for your time. I know this was difficult for you to make it on my show. I really appreciate it, and I look forward to speaking with you in the future. Thank you so much.

Dr. Paul:　　I look forward to it as well. Thank you, Joel.

Dr. Gould:　　Great. We'll talk to you soon. Okay, everybody. This is the end of my half hour radio show. I hope it was at least a little bit informative. I can't be any more passionate about my new cause, sleep disorders. There's other topics we're going to discuss, but it's something that I'm going to fall back on, and I'm really curious and excited, because one of the things that Dr. Paul is going to be doing for me is he's going to be tracking my physical health after I get treated for this.

I still haven't gotten my Mandibular Advancement Device, and I literally wake up in the morning now thinking, how much did I sleep? Should I do another sleep study? Did I get any restful sleep? I'm really excited to see. Through me we're going to follow what my blood pressure does and see is there any physical changes? I'm hoping I'm going to grow hair back, but that might be asking too much. I shared with you also before that I do have something called Crohn's disease, which is an autoimmune disease, and we'll discuss how that might actually be affected by sleep apnea.

I want to say, please remember prevention is everything. All dentistry is cosmetic. You got to feel good from the inside out. Thanks for listening. I want to thank my producer, Mario DiGiovanni. You're the best. Everybody, until next week, see you soon. Get your smile on and be well.

GYSO – Eps. 4
Dr. Patti Panucci Orthodontics

Dr. Gould: Hello, welcome to Wednesday night at 7:00PM. This is Dr. Joel Gould. You are listening to my show called Get Your Smile On. This, as I always promise, is going to be the most exciting half hour radio show on dentistry that can be found. Tonight I'm pretty excited to bring you one of my favorite orthodontists around town, Dr. Patti Panucci, and we will get to her later. I just want to reintroduce myself to everybody. I am the wellness dentist. You can think of it this way, prevention is wellness. If we can catch a problem before it gets too big, you will be much happier. You'll save time. You'll save money, and you will save pain and aggravation.

Tonight what I want to talk about is, first of all I'm the founder of Modern American Dentistry, and the acronym is MAD. What I'm doing is trying to bring dentistry into the modern age. A lot of what I want to talk about has to do with the whole person rather than just focusing on the teeth. As I said last week, the eyes are the window to the soul. The oral cavity is the gateway to the rest of the body. Last week we spoke with the incredible Dr. Paul Knittel about his emergency location in Redondo Beach, and we talked about some medical and dental emergencies that would require an urgent trip to the hospital.

Modern American Dentistry, for me, stands for updating, simplifying, and making dentistry easy, removing the barriers to having a great smile and feeling good. Today I want to talk to you about a really important topic, and that is modernizing orthodontics. What are orthodontics? What is orthodontics? Orthodontia actually comes from the Greek word *orthos* 'to correct or straight'. When we combine it with *dontia* which is the Greek word for 'teeth' we have orthodontia. To simplify it, we're going to talk about straightening teeth.

Apparently the specialty of orthodontics, and it is a separate specialty in dentistry, is one of the first dental specialties in existence. There are apparently mummies that have been found that are over 2,000 years old that have bands on their teeth. That's not a joke. In ancient Egypt dentistry was a pretty big business. I wonder what going to the early orthodontist would have cost, and I guess you paid with a goat or a chicken or gold coins. I can't really say. Interesting, the source that orthodontics is the first dental specialty came from Wikipedia, and when are they ever wrong?

Some people will say, "I don't care about my teeth. Why bother? As long as I can chew, I'm fine." Having straight teeth really isn't just for looks. Aligned teeth wear better. Aligned teeth have healthier gums. When your teeth are crowded plaque and all the terrible things that we've discussed in the past about not flossing have an easier way to get into the tissue supporting your teeth. So we definitely want to be thinking about the healthful reasons why we'd want to have straight teeth.

Now I'm going to talk about a lot of things on this podcast that have to do with science and humans and evolution, and I really want to go on record as saying there are three topics that you never talk about in a dental office, and those are sex, religion, and politics. I want to preface this by saying I truly believe that all religions are just fantastic, and people who believe in them and who are from those particular religions I know bring such a great source of comfort to people. I think it's fantastic. Now my views of evolution, they do not conflict with views on religion. I think that that's sort of come more to the forefront these days. Scientifically speaking a lot of the dental things we're going to talk about have an evolutionary cause or beginning.

Let's get into orthodontics. Straight teeth, they're healthier in general. How do we do this? How do we move teeth around in the jaw? How could that even work? When we put pressure on a tooth in any direction what we get is the osteoclasts, which are the cells that will dissolve bone if we put pressure in one direction. As those osteoclasts eat up the bone and let the tooth move forward, different cells called osteoblasts produce new bone behind the tooth so that as a tooth moves forward through the gums we don't have the tooth drifting around and not being steady. It's very important to understand that when it comes to orthodontics it doesn't really matter what type of braces that you're going to put on. It could be a removable appliance. It could be old-school metal braces. Whatever we're going to do with our teeth, they're going to moved by pressure that we place.

Once we get the teeth into the ideal position, then we're going to want to hold them in that place, and that's called retention. That's where the name for a retainer comes from. When you're finished with your orthodontics you get your braces taken off, and you have to wear your retainers. That's to make sure that the cellular changes that all of these osteoclasts and osteoblasts have done to move your teeth into that ideal position that gets solidified, and that those tissues get to mature and stay in one place.

The interesting thing about orthodontics is that when you move a tooth through bone it brings the gums and everything with it. That's a very interesting topic when it comes to having wear on teeth. As you wear away a tooth it continues to erupt into your mouth, but not just the tooth. It brings with it the gums and the bone. So you will see occasionally, hopefully not too often around my office, somebody who has that gummy smile where their teeth have been worn down, and they show a lot of gums. This can actually be over or excessive orthodontic movement.

How can the average American look better than Tom Cruise, Gwen Stefani, and Beyoncé? The answer is clear. Those people in the entertainment industry they did not opt for clear aligners. Clear aligners, such as Invisalign and Clear Correct, are systems of clear aligners that a patient will change out every two weeks until the orthodontic treatment is complete. This has revolutionized orthodontics, and it's pretty incredible. The American Orthodontic Association and American Dental Association made a note that over the past 15 years the increase in orthodontics being done on people in America has gone up 58%. That's a huge jump, but this increase just so happens to coincide with the FDA's approval of clear aligners as orthodontic treatment. I don't think it's any coincidence. People who've had braces before, they know all the pitfalls and all the issues that come with those old-school metal brackets.

I wanted to really clear away all the beginning parts of talking about orthodontics, and I want to make sure that when we get Dr. Panucci on that she can get to the most interesting and exciting new developments in orthodontics, rather than talking about the boring stuff like, why would we move teeth and how do teeth move? I'm a systems guy. I'm a formula guy, and I do a great TV segment on clear aligners, and I have a clear formula. These are the reasons why clear aligners are in a lot of cases better than metal braces. Clear aligners can actually move teeth almost completely as successfully as fixed braces, but there are definitely some limitations. However, when treatment is done properly the results will be exactly the same as regular old-school metal braces.

People always want to ask, should this be a lot cheaper? The answer is technically it is and it isn't. It's still fairly expensive. What we do with clear aligners is, and getting back to my formula, the C in the clear stands for Custom. These aligners are custom made for you by a computer program from impressions taken from your mouth. Regular metal braces come out of a box, and your orthodontist has to put them on your teeth and put in different wires to move the teeth in directions that we want them to move. What's so great about the clear aligners is that they're custom made just for each and every person.

The L in clear stands for Lips. These clear aligners are really comfortable. When you get metal braces or ceramic braces those are very sharp, and they'll cut your lips up quite a bit until you get comfortable. When I had them on I actually couldn't tolerate them. I'm a bit of a baby when it comes to dental procedures myself, and I had Dr. Panucci take my regular braces off, and she did some Invisalign on me instead. We'll be talking to her about that in just a few minutes. The L in the clear formula is for lips, so your lips really don't get cut.

The E stands for Easy. You just pop them into your mouth. You don't have to spend time at the orthodontist having them cemented. The A stands for Access. You can pop them out, brush, floss, and put them right back in. That is a huge advantage to anybody who's had braces recently who knows how messy and how much food can get caught in those braces. The R in the clear formula stand for Removable, the most obvious one. These aligners are so incredible. If you have a big night out or a speaking engagement you simply pop them out of your mouth and leave them at home. You can't do that with regular braces.

Tonight I am excited to bring to you Dr. Patti Panucci. We're going to get to her in a couple seconds here. I just want to let everybody know that she's a graduate of the University of Louisville in Kentucky, and she graduated with a DMD, that's a Doctor of Medical Dentistry. It's different than a DDS, but we're both dentists. She attended one of the top ranked orthodontic schools in America, University of South California, for her graduate program. That's pretty impressive. She is a member of the Pacific Coast Society of Orthodontists, the West LA Dental Society, California Dental Association. She speaks for the American Association of Orthodontists and a whole bunch of other great associations. She's a regular contributor to the community, and she's a great person who does a lot of charity work. I can't think of a better guest to have on my show.

I'm going to go to a commercial in just a second, and when I come back I hope to have for you the lovely and fantastic Patti Panucci.

All right, everybody. Welcome back. Thank you for listening. You are listening to Get Your Smile On with Dr. Joel Gould. Tonight's guest is the, speaking of modern dentistry, she is a pretty modern lady when it comes to orthodontics. We're welcoming the wonderful Dr. Patti Panucci. Are you there?

Dr. Patti:	I am here. Can you hear me all right?
Dr. Gould:	I can hear you just great.
Dr. Patti:	Excellent. Thank you for having me.

Dr. Gould: My pleasure. I'm so excited to have you on. I know you're going to be on my show more than once. First of all, you're a captivating speaker. You know what you're talking about, and that's really important stuff that I want to get out there to the general public talking about early airway development and exactly when to bring your child to the orthodontist, and all the problems that we've talked about regarding sleep disorders. We'll get to that a little later. Today I really wanted to introduce you to all of my listeners, and I wanted the opportunity to have you say a few things about what orthodontics have become. I talked about, prior to you being on the show, I got the nuts and bolts of dentistry out of the way, so you wouldn't have to talk about osteoblasts and osteoclasts. I really want to just talk to you about what's new and what's out there. The first question I really want to ask you is what do you love about your work? What is it about orthodontics that makes you happy?

Dr. Patti: Of course, I love my patients. I love watching the kids grow up and getting to know the adults over the course of treatment. Many of them are very interesting, have awesome jobs. What really is fun is learning challenging ways to help patients accomplish and obtain that beautiful smile that they want. There's so many new aesthetic treatments out there, and technology is rapidly changing in orthodontics, so it's really fun to keep up with all the new technology.

Dr. Gould: Great, and that's what I really wanted to talk about today. I wanted to first ask you, I know that you do a lot of Invisalign, and I did talk about what clear aligners are and all that. Orthodontics are specialists, so general dentists do some minor orthodontics, some do a little more, but what's the most popular treatment that you do at your office?

Dr. Patti: Definitely that would be Invisalign. I have over 40% of my patients in some sort of clear aligner treatment, the majority in Invisalign. It's very easy, and they love it. You can get just as great results as with traditional brackets and wires.

Dr. Gould: That's the information that I have as well. I want to talk more about, for the Invisalign and the clear aligners, I know that you are a high level provider for the teen version of this. I really want you to sort of explain about what's different about an adult who's going to get some Invisalign versus a teenager or somebody who's still developing. What would you say to somebody who said, why can't my regular dentist do this for my 11 year old?

Dr. Patti: Sure. The teen product for Invisalign has been out for several years now, and I have been treating quite a few teens with it. I think what comes with orthodontists as a specialty is we're not just tooth movers. We're also jaw analyzers.

Dr. Gould: No pressure, Patti. This is only live. It's okay. I've messed up a few things. That's part of the fun of being on radio. It's good. I like it. Why not?

Dr. Patti: We're looking at the big picture, so orthotics isn't just about moving the teeth. It's assessing the jaw growth, and in teens that's definitely what's happening. We can influence the direction of the jaw growth, and orthopedics is a part of the specialty. It's orthodontics and dentofacial orthopedics. That training isn't delivered in dental school for general dentists. It's that extra 2-3 years that the orthodontist go through to gain the training in the orthopedic portion of treatment. So that's why it really would be great to have an orthodontist treat a growing patient as opposed to a general dentist.

Dr. Gould: So you brought to light all the important reasons why I agree with you. What people don't always think about is when you do these different appliances, we want to call them devices, because an appliance is a stove or fridge, but when we do these and the child is growing these are, especially with the clear aligners, they're rigid. So as this child is growing it could actually even stunt their growth or the growth or expansion of their jaw. What age would you think, we're going to get to talking a little bit about airway development, but for a regular orthodontic case for a teen Invisalign, somebody that you feel has a great airway and is a good candidate, what age would you want to start that patient at? How long would this type of treatment take, on average?

Dr. Patti: On average the typical teenager will have a full set of their adult teeth around age 12 or 13. That would be an ideal time where we still have the opportunity to use the time that they're still growing to gain some of that orthopedic change I was mentioning earlier. The idea age would be about 12 or 13. An average treatment time at that age, it definitely varies on the complexity of the case, but anywhere from 12-24 months.

Dr. Gould: I'm thinking back to my childhood, and I had headgear, and I had all that stuff. The whole idea behind headgear is to help with development as the child grows. Is there a comparable type of thing that you do with Invisalign? We don't have to get graphic if it's too intense, but it's just something that you would do to stabilize somebody in a different way, because we don't have the old-school brackets?

Dr. Patti: Absolutely. When patients and doctors think of Invisalign they'll think simply the clear aligners, but there are many devices, like you mentioned earlier, that we can use in conjunction with the clear aligners to obtain the results that we want, the orthopedic change, as well as additional tooth movement. Axillaries, as I call them, can be applied as well. Headgear is more of an old-school type of device, but there are many new more user friendly, patient friendly.

Dr. Gould: Now Patti, wait a second, my orthodontist when I was 12 or 13 years old, he insisted that I wear my high pull headgear to school every day. I don't anybody who's listening, high pull headgear—

Dr. Patti: I'm sorry.

Dr. Gould: I know, right? It's pretty crazy. You just made me feel very old. Part of my whole conversation about dentistry is wanting to modernize it, so that's sort of my mandate is bringing dentistry into the modern age. I think that you really set me straight on that. Technology's really changed, and there are better ways then to embarrass a child or make them feel even more uncomfortable at that age. There you go.

Dr. Patti: Absolutely.

Dr. Gould: I know that some people they're not good with clear aligners. What's funny is with me I know we went through the reverse that most people go through. I thought I'm going to get metal braces, or ceramic braces, and it's going to be faster, and it's going to be easier. Then I was pretty miserable. I've already admitted that I'm not the greatest patient, and you ended up taking off my braces. I'm sorry to do that to you. You're very kind not to give me too hard of a time. I know that you have some other types of fixed brackets that are more appropriate for people who really aren't a good candidate or don't want to do clear aligners. I know that you specialize in a couple of different more aesthetic or more cosmetic treatments. Can you tell us more about that?

Dr. Patti: Sure thing. A lot of patients will think that maybe the Invisalign is a bit of a burden in some sort of sense with keeping track of the aligners, removing them during eating. An alternative is braces behind the teeth. We call those lingual braces, because they're on the inside, the tongue side, which in anatomy is called the lingual side. That's why they're called the lingual braces. They're very aesthetic. You can't see them at all. They're used to accomplish the same results that we would with clear aligners or braces on the outside of the teeth.

Dr. Gould: That's great. I'm sure a lot of people listening wouldn't really have thought of that. That's a really great idea. Is it tougher to choose who's appropriate, or is it pretty easy that almost you can put them on anybody?

Dr. Patti: No, because they are behind the teeth, you think about how your teeth come together, the lower teeth definitely have to be behind the upper teeth. There are certain instances where it wouldn't be ideal for a patient to have those. If the upper teeth cover the bottom teeth significantly then they'd be in a situation where we'd need to prop their bite open, which could be uncomfortable.

Dr. Gould: Right.

Dr. Patti: So there are definitely some cases that are more appropriate than others.

Dr. Gould: Okay. That gets me to the next point here. Basically somebody should really see an orthodontist if they need to have some orthodontics done. I want to talk about you, your location. You are in beautiful Manhattan Beach. How can people get a hold of you? Tell me what your website is. I know, but I want my listeners to hear.

Dr. Patti: Sure. The best way, go to my website. It's BeachBraces. org. You can request an appointment online there. It will give you our phone number, feel free to call. We have every sort of social media platform out there, Twitter, Facebook, Instagram. You definitely can find us online.

Dr. Gould: You just made my job easier. I was going to ask you about social media. I know that you are one of the dentists who's embraced it for exactly what it is, and you've been doing it right from the start. So people can follow you on Facebook, and they can watch what you've got going on at the office.

Dr. Patti: Yeah. It's been really fun. It's been great. We get to show before and after smiles on there, highlight some of the new technology that you and I just talked about. It's been really interactive and fun.

Dr. Gould: Excellent. You just made me remember. I know that when the kids get their braces taken off they get to have a picture taken. My Invisalign is pretty much done, so I'm looking forward to having my picture taken, and I can post it on social media. What do you do for kids who finish with their braces?

Dr. Patti: They get to wear the famous crown.

Dr. Gould: I can't wait.

Dr. Patti: We'll give you a picture, and of course we'll give you lots of goodies. Our patients who have had braces for a long period of time are supposed to stay away from certain foods, so we always like to give them those, hard, sticky, crunchy things. We definitely do a little celebration, and it's a fun moment to unveil the smile and celebrate the office.

Dr. Gould: I can't wait. I know all of your people there, and I always come in and give everybody a hard time. So I'm looking forward to when I come in and get my photo done with the crown. I want to sort of wind things down here, but I want to talk about something that's really important. I've mentioned this is a couple of my other shows. It's something that is such a major topic that I'm going to definitely be utilizing every opportunity I have to speak about this, and these are sleep disordered breathing. You and I have talked about this in depth, and we talked about the changes. Just real briefly, suggestions. We're going to go into this in greater detail, but I know that traditionally people are wanting to send their kids to the orthodontist a little later. What do you think? When do you like to see a child to assess the formation of an airway to make sure that we have proper growth, and when do you think that you as an orthodontist could start to get in there and have some affect?

Dr. Patti: The American Association of Orthodontist recommends that all children be seen by age 7 for an orthodontic evaluation. We can definitely intervene even earlier than that if a pediatrician or physician would see the need. Definitely by age 7 I think every single child should have a screening. You can analyze the growth, analyze the jaw growth, the airway, and it's a key time to get that evaluation.

Dr. Gould: I really wanted people to understand that we don't wait till age 12 or 13 to start putting braces on adult teeth, and we're going to be talking about the formation of the airway. I'm going to have a lot of different people talking about this. It's such a huge topic. I want to just take the opportunity to thank you and welcome you to my show. I really look forward to having you back when we can get into a little more specifics on this huge topic of sleep disordered breathing. I really look forward to it.

Dr. Patti: Thank you. Thank you for having me. It was very fun. I look forward to speaking with everyone again.

Dr. Gould: Awesome. Thank you, Patti. Have a great night. We'll see you soon.

That was Dr. Patti Panucci, and she's such a great spokesperson for her profession. I really love it. We are really going to talk about a lot of airway and breathing disorders. I really want to make them as interesting and exciting as they should be, considering that so few people know really what's affecting their breathing in their sleep and their airway. We'll get to that soon.

Today we're just about out of time. I want to thank my producer, Maria DiGiovanni, and anybody can follow us on SoundCloud under Dr. Joel Gould, soon to be on iTunes. You can also follow us under Modern American Dentistry on Facebook. I believe we've got our Instagram account going, and I look forward to having some really great before and after instant fixes of cosmetic dentistry, and remember, all dentistry is cosmetic. I'd just like to say thank you to all my listeners. I look forward to bringing you all the latest, greatest, most exciting information in the world of dentistry. Remember that prevention is wellness. Thank you for listening to my show on wellness dentistry. We'll see you soon. Thank you.

GYSO – Eps. 5
Dr. Steven Park Sleep Medicine

Dr. Gould: All right, everybody, welcome to Get Your Smile On. I am Dr. Joel Gould, your wellness dentist, and what we have for you tonight is the most exciting half hour podcast on dentistry and wellness dentistry in the world. I'm going to say that, make that claim, and I'd like somebody to prove me wrong.

Last week we had the exciting and very communicative Dr. Patti Panucci. We talked about orthodontics, and we will get her back on the show soon. She's fantastic. Tonight's topic, I've talked about this a few times before, and this a really huge topic. So tonight we're going to be discussing something that nobody wants to hear about. What I want to talk about is what do we need to live? We need three things. We need food, water, and air. Obviously we need a lot more than that, like PlayStations and Xbox and wine and walks along the beach, but we can live for three weeks without food. We can live for three days without water. We can only live for three minutes without air.

We spend one third of our lives sleeping. We know what we do the two thirds of the time that we're not sleeping, but the information that's come to me very recently about myself, about many people, is that for one third of our life we no idea what's going on. Today's topic of discussion is sleep disordered breathing. I have a personal story with this, because I admitted last week or the week before that I have obstructive sleep apnea.

Sleep disordered breathing isn't just obstructive sleep apnea. It is also something that's much lesser known, but just as serious, upper airway resistance syndrome, or UARS. This is the sister version to obstructive sleep apnea, and what's different about this is this isn't the type of person that you'd expect when you think of sleep apnea. I know people think a heavy guy with a big neck who snores really loud. That's your sleep apnea person. What I've come to find very recently is that that's completely untrue. Many people suffer from different sleep disorders related to breathing, and nobody can know who they are until we actually test and find out.

Tonight I'm going to be discussing this topic in detail with my guest, who is an ENT medical doctor and sleep doctor. We'll be bringing him on very shortly, because he's got a lot of information that we want to talk about.

A couple of different things I want to talk about here. We talked about oxygen. Everyone has an ideal oxygen saturation rate, and that's a fancy way for saying when you breathe the amount of oxygen that goes on to your blood should be a certain percentage. Ideal would be 98%. That'd be great. If you hold your breath for as long as you can you cannot get your oxygen levels to drop below about 93, 94, but I'd say probably you couldn't get it to go down more than 1 or 2%. When someone is sleeping and their oxygen drops down by at least 4% this is a very serious thing. That 4% drop in oxygen signals to your body that you are choking. You're not breathing.

What happens? Your body has a reaction that we've all heard about, fight or flight. What happens with fight or flight? Your hormones go crazy. Your body thinks that you're dying, and your heart rate increases. Your body wakes you up. You wake up out of sleep over and over again all night long. That type of activity you think that you'd notice, but most people don't. It's very little known, and I had no idea either. I thought I was a great sleeper. If you would have asked me, "Do you know what sleep apnea is?" I would have said with anyone else, "Not me, I don't have it. I'm fine. I sleep great. I don't snore." Boy, was I wrong. Not only was I wrong, but I was so wrong that I didn't realize just how seriously this was affecting me.

Why is this so important? This is an epidemic. This is one of the largest public health issues affecting all of Western medicine all around the world. Sleep is very important. Just on a basic level, because we will cover this in a different podcast, sleep is important for so many reasons. It's the one time during your life that you actually let your brain sort itself out. We get into our REM sleep, and it lets your body start to heal. Only in the deep stages of sleep does your body truly and fully emit all the hormones and all the chemical mediators that you need to live and be healthy.

I want to get right to my guest tonight, because I want to discuss this. There's so many interesting things that have to do with this. Tonight my guest is Dr. Steven Park. He is board certified in sleep medicine, and he is board certified ENT including head and neck surgery. He received his undergraduate degree from John's Hopkins and his medical degree from Columbia. He took his ENT fellowship at Einstein Montefiore, and I had to look that one up, but I want to ask Dr. Park about that in one second. He is also the author of a #1 New York Times bestselling book called *Sleep Interrupted*, and he reveals the number one reason why many of us are sick and tired. He's got another book that's coming out that is called *The Complete Guide to Getting the Sleep You Need For the Life You Want*. Dr. Park, are you on the line?\

Dr. Park: I'm here.

Dr. Gould:	Great to have you on my show. Thank you so much. You're on the East Coast. How is everything going over there in New York?
Dr. Park:	It's very nice and cool.
Dr. Gould:	I like it. This is the time of year where you have a lot of humidity.
Dr. Park:	Yes. That just broke earlier today. It's very pleasant right now.
Dr. Gould:	Great. That's good. California we're having some humidity come in this weekend, and everybody's already panicking. It might actually be a little bit damp. Dr. Park I want to let you just tell us a little bit about your fellowship. I looked up Montefiore, and it's a pretty special school. Do you want to tell us sort of what's unique about it?
Dr. Park:	Sure. Actually the sleep lab at Montefiore was one of the first places where they had sleep technicians, and it was one of the pioneering sleep labs for development of the field of sleep apnea and sleep medicine. Let me just clarify a couple of things. My book was not a New York Times #1 bestseller. I wish it were. It was endorsed by numerous New York Times bestselling authors. That's one of my goals eventually.
Dr. Gould:	Trust me on this. When everybody listens to this podcast and goes and orders it it may get to #1 on the New York Times bestselling list.
Dr. Park:	I hope so.
Dr. Gould:	Great. Sorry about that. Thank you for correcting me.
Dr. Park:	Also, I'm board certified in otolaryngology, which is ENT, and also sleep medicine.
Dr. Gould:	Great. Sorry about that. I guess this is new for me. I've listened to your podcast, and you have your lovely wife who helps you out. I've got my producer who's behind

the scenes, and she's great, but I'm getting used to being able to speak in an appropriate way. Sometimes I'm going to mess up, but I do apologize.

Dr. Park: No problem whatsoever.

Dr. Gould: I guess we should probably talk about you. It's a very unusual combination, or for most people who don't understand what sleep and breathing disorders are it's unusual. What can you tell us? What brought you to this career path?

Dr. Park: I was in general otolaryngology in head and neck surgery for 13 years before I came to Montefiore four years ago. When I was in private practice in Manhattan I was doing a lot of sinus surgery, routine stuff that most ENTs did, and a lot of ear, nose, and throat medicine and surgery. One thing that I noticed was that whenever I did sinus surgery for the most part they did well, but for about 10-20% of the patients they kept coming back with recurrent symptoms. Almost invariably, we actually did a study showing that about 80% of these patients had undiagnosed sleep apnea. So then when I started looking for sleep apnea before I started doing sinus surgery, many patients didn't need sinus surgery. They got much better. That just kind of opened my eyes to the possibility that the sleep breathing disorders were an underlying problem with many of these chronic conditions, not just with ear, nose, and throat conditions, but pretty much every chronic condition out there in medicine.

Dr. Gould: You just said a huge mouthful. This is really only a couple of years ago then, so this isn't something that is widely known. This is something that you noticed, and then you said this is something I want to investigate further. Did you get any sort of pushback from your colleagues over what was going on?

Dr. Park: Before I started doing that, before I wrote my book, I started to look at all the research out there, and what I found was that if you obstruct, and if you have reflux, because those two go hand in hand, every time you obstruct you bring up your stomach juices into your throat. That can cause more swelling and then more obstructions. It's a vicious cycle. One aggravates the other. Then that leads into more inflammation in the ears, nose, and throat, the lungs, causing sinus infections, ear infections, asthma, bronchitis, and then that causes further obstruction, causing low levels of oxygen like what you were talking about. There are research studies linking every one of these points, connecting the dots. I made this huge diagram that I described in my book, where all these chronic conditions are linked to sleeping and breathing problems and reflux.

Dr. Gould: We're at 2015. Were you kind of surprised that you had to figure this out on your own, that nobody else had sort of put the pieces of the puzzle together?

Dr. Park: I'm not the only one to do this. The problem is that there are many people who have been talking about these concepts for many years, but there's really no one mainstream organization that really promotes these kind of ideas, because everyone has their own agenda. I had to go a little bit outside of medicine, especially within the dental fields, especially with their emphasis on craniofacial jaw development. I remember there's one of my mentors who passed away a few years ago, Dr. Brian Palmer. I don't know if you know who he is, but he kind of enlightened me to the possibilities that the physical act of bottle feeding can aggravate malocclusion. He has lots of studies and papers that he produced showing that that's the case. That kind of led me to learn that the way you use your mouth as a child, also as an adult, can affect the way your jaw develops, and if your jaws don't develop fully then your airway gets more narrow.

Dr. Gould: Right. It's very obvious to me as a dentist when I'm shining a light onto people's mouths all day long that I'm seeing their mouth and their throat, and I think I shared this with you. This is my 25th year in practice, and I have been treating people with bruxism with brux guards or with grinding guards, and it's successful. So I was one of those people who was missing the diagnosis. I saw a symptom, and I treated the symptom, and I do one heck of a good brux guard, but it's just putting a Band-Aid on the greater issue, and that's sleep and sleep disordered breathing issues.

To me, when I got into this, and I started this a couple years ago. We do a lot of continuing education, and I was kind of fascinated by the idea that dentists would be involved in treating sleep problems. It wasn't until very recently that I myself was diagnosed with obstructive sleep apnea that this became so important to me. I hate to be one of those people that has to experience it themselves before they really truly understand. I think I kind of had that same moment as you where I saw the pieces of the puzzle that were sitting directly in front of me the whole time, but I never put them together in the right way.

What brought you to go to dentists? We talked about the development, the craniofacial development. Is there an orthodontic school of thought that you've gotten used to working with?

Dr. Paul: Honestly, from what I can tell it's not mainstream dentistry. A lot of the concepts go completely against traditional orthodontics and dentistry, including the concept of how teeth get straightened. Ultimately the focus amongst these rogue dentists, so to speak, are they focus on the airway, pure and simple. That starts from early childhood development. You can even say that it starts within the mother's womb.

Dr. Gould: What factors would be in the womb? Would that be certain factors that we're talking about, mostly nutrition and Vitamin D and that? Is there anything that you know that in that stage would lead towards this type of a problem?

Dr. Paul: First of all, if the mother is susceptible to sleep breathing problems, then that's going to aggravate sleep apnea during pregnancy, and we know that that's a huge epidemic amongst pregnant women that's not being treated at all. So any degree of physiologic stress can prevent problem development of the baby. We also know that prematurity, which is another huge epidemic these days, prematurity has been shown to be a major risk factor for sleep apnea development in the future.

Dr. Gould: That's incredible.

Dr. Paul: Also if you add the obesity epidemic we know that if you're overweight that's going to significantly raise your risk of sleep apnea, and if you're pregnant that's a double whammy.

Dr. Gould: Right. As I sort of delve into this topic, because it's so far-reaching I was saying, when I understood the enormity of this problem it made me really confused that the medical field, the medical industry, hasn't put more pieces together and said, we should at least look into this. Do you feel sometimes that you're sort of screaming at the top of your lungs, but nobody's listening?

Dr. Paul: Yes. That's one of the reasons why I started to reach out to the public. I wrote my book, and I started this blog, and I write and I speak. One of my main missions, besides helping patients one to one, is to reach out to the public and educate the general public so that they can be empowered to know what's going on. Many of these patients, or not even my patients, but people who ready my blog and read my book, they actually are educating their doctors as to what's going on.

Dr. Gould: Right. We've already experienced that. I've had some patients who, now that I'm aware of this I've been reviewing people's medical history. I had a guy in today 33 years old, and we take a blood pressure on anybody that we're going to be doing anesthetic on. When I saw his blood pressure, I looked at him, and I said, "You're a pretty fit guy. Why do you have high blood pressure?" He said, "I don't know, but my doctor wants to put me on high blood pressure medication." I thought, what are the chances that I'm so focused on this? I tipped him back, and I looked in his mouth, and he has all of the usual signs that I have recently learned are an indicator that this person mostly likely has an issue with sleep apnea.

He had a scalloped tongue, which is when your tongue is pushing up against your teeth. It takes on the shape of the teeth. He had inflamed tonsils and a large uvula. I said to him, "Do you snore?" He said, "I snore really loudly. My wife makes me sleep in the other room." I said, "Did your doctor at any point in time suggest that maybe you should get checked or tested for sleep apnea?" He said, "Absolutely not," but then he went further to say, "I think I have it." He gave me a couple different reasons. I thought, how incredible is this that, we're not in a backwater town here. This is Los Angeles, and medical doctors it's not that they're not getting it, they're not even asking the question.

Dr. Paul: I actually have a very similar story. Many years ago I had a friend who lived very close to me. He had recurrent sinus infections, and he was going to his ENT for many years. He suspected that he may have sleep apnea, so he kept bringing this up to his doctor. The doctor said, "You don't fit the profile. You definitely don't have sleep apnea." This went on for many years. Eventually we became friends, and I ended up diagnosing him with a sleep study with sever sleep apnea. Then he started to sleep much better using a C-PAP. It just goes to show that there's a lot of misconceptions and stereotypes amongst even mainstream doctors that still think that you have to fit this typical profile, and I think one thing that you and I both bring up often is that you don't have to fit the particular profile. You can be young, thin, even not a snorer and still have severe sleep apnea.

Dr. Gould: Right. That's something that really is kind of blowing my mind, because for myself when I look back and I see all the medical issues that I've had they all could be attributed to sleep apnea, and it all makes perfect sense. I wouldn't have seen it until I saw one thing that changed my life, and that was seeing my sleep study. When I came back after seeing that sleep study to my office I started just to casually ask questions, because I know what my perception of sleep apnea was.

So the things I would ask, I would say, "Have you been tested for sleep apnea?" Right away people would say, "Not me, I don't have it." I wanted to say, and these are my patients so I don't want to be hard on them, but I wanted to say, "I didn't ask you if you had it. I asked you if you were tested." There seems to be a huge perception that, first of all, not me, I don't have it, it's somebody else. What do you think has brought on this, it's almost like when I ask somebody, and of course I don't ask that anymore, because it's almost insulting. I think people get literally insulted that you would even ask them. Is it an assumption that you're saying they're fat or not healthy? They take it so seriously. J

Dr. Park: I think that there is some component of being embarrassed, because if you have sleep apnea then, again, even the public has a stereotype that you have to be heavy, overweight, snore, and have a big neck. So they don't want to be lumped into that crowd. Some people just don't know that they have a problem, because they perceive that they're sleeping well.

Dr. Gould: Again, I was one of those people. We talked earlier, as a wellness dentist, and I could define what wellness dentistry is, and even some of my best friends are like, what are yo talking about? Discussing what wellness is in someone's overall health is you can't say to the dentist, "You just deal with the teeth and nothing else." You at a very early stage realized that if you're dealing with the airway you're going to have to start to talk to the people that deal with that, and that's dentists. When you first became aware that we could something called a mandibular advancement device or a MAD, was that really shocking? Was there a lot of stuff out there? What gave you the idea that you really wanted to work on this further working with dentists?

Dr. Park: If you look at the evolution of sleep apnea treatment, before 1980 all we had was a tracheotomy where we put a hole in your neck into your windpipe. Then C-PAP was developed and the palate operation was developed around the early 80s. Even the mandibular advancement devices there were prototypes that were being described in that same timeframe. For whatever reason the dental appliances never took off as quickly as C-PAP or surgical options. It's been around for a really long time, but I think even when

I was in private practice about 10 years ago it wasn't really that well known about or even popular.

I think one of the major impediments was just accessibility, because most insurance companies weren't covering it. That's changed 180 degrees where most insurances do cover it, and many dentists are taking insurance. Even people are just more aware, so they'll pay cash, and they'll pay what it takes to sleep better. There's been this dramatic increase in awareness by the public and also sleep physicians and medical doctors about usefulness of these dental appliances.

Dr. Gould: Right. I listened to your podcast on MADs, mandibular advancement devices, and it was pretty great. What I wanted to get to, and the biggest thing about this topic is when you mention sleep apnea everyone thinks of that C-PAP machine, the giant mask. It's been only a couple of years, about 5 years, that the MAD would be considered the equivalent for moderate and mild sleep apnea. I now that the studies are there, but it's fairly recent.

Dr. Park: Yeah. Those are an accumulation of numerous large scale studies. When the American Academy of sleep medicine puts out these position statements they have hundreds of studies and pick the best ones. They don't say these things lightly. There's strong evidence now that these devices are equivalent to C-PAP for people with mild to moderate sleep apnea. A little caveat though. It doesn't get the numbers down as low as C-PAP, but in general people will tolerate and use the oral appliances for longer periods of time, so basically it's a wash.

Dr. Gould: Some of the stats that I heard was that only 3% of everyone in America is being properly treated for sleep apnea, and that makes perfect sense, because a lot of people get their C-PAP machine. They put it on Craig-

slist. They put it in their closet. They stuff it away somewhere, because it's about as unsexy as you can get. Not
that a mandibular advancement device is sexy. Again,
I see a lot of people with bruxism, and these are people
who are wearing something in their mouth anyway. So
they already have their protocol where they'll brush
their teeth, and they'll get ready for bed, and they'll
put this device in. So it's something that's just so much
easier, especially if you travel too.

We're getting close to the end of our time here, but
there's still so many questions I want to ask you. What
I want my listeners to understand is we can talk about
sleep apnea and this and that, but I listened to some of
your podcasts, and there's really some compelling stuff.
What I would like you to do, you have the opportunity to speak to my listeners and say, what are the top 3
things that we're really worried about with sleep apnea?
Why is this such a big deal?

Before I let you do that what I wanted to actually say
was that I'm excited that the medical insurance companies have been smart enough to realize that getting
someone treated for an internal device is going to be
in the long run so much cheaper than treating them
for so many medications and procedures and surgeries.
They've recognized that this is definitely a cost effective
measure to treat this. I think that it's such a huge step
forward. I'm technically impressed. Medical insurance
companies, they just want to save money. We hope they
care about us too.

What would you say? I do want to scare my patients,
because if they don't take this seriously this is something that's really major, and just seeing the reduction
in my health recently because this has come up so
quickly. What would you say to scare people, but real-

istically? We talked about brain damage. When you get brain damage, how does it happen? Maybe you want to start there.

Dr. Park: That's a huge topic. Topics that I've had in the past on my podcast on memory loss and brain damage those are some of the most popular, most reviewed. There's tons of research in the scientific literature on the detrimental effects of sleep apnea and low oxygen levels on brain function and development. There's more and more cross talking between the sleep apnea researchers and the dementia researchers these days. There's this huge overlap that's not being explored. You think that Alzheimer's is a different condition than sleep apnea brain damage, but if you look at the mechanisms it's probably the same. There are ongoing studies now that are looking at this issue. Clinically on a daily basis I see patients who have obvious undiagnosed sleep apnea for decades, and they clearly have memory loss, mild cognitive impairment and early dementia. It's a scary problem.

Dr. Gould: What's funny is that you know so much about this, and when I read your mission statement on your website, which I actually wanted to let everybody that your website is DrStevenPark.com, and you're easy to find. DrStevenPark.com, and we'll have your link up on our site at some point in time here. On your website anybody can go and listen to your different discussions on brain damage and all these other things that sleep apnea is causing. What do you think? It's 2015, and I saw a lot of stuff from five years ago of dentists trying to bring this up more to the public, and we weren't ready. When do you think that the moment the tipping point? What do you see coming up that's really going to be what actually gets all medical doctors to take a step back and say, I don't know everything about this. Maybe I should listen. Do you think we're close?

Dr. Park: I'm a little bit pessimistic. The problem is that the health-care system is so overwhelmed already, financially and in terms of the volume of people who need services. The problem is that sleep services there's such a huge demand, and not enough supply of sleep services. To get a sleep study in some parts of the country it can be weeks or months. It's really frustrating even in a major metropolitan area, for me, to get patients to undergo sleep studies. With home testing I think that's going to be changing. Many insurance companies are requiring home tests as first line diagnostic tools for routine, run of the mill, sleep apnea patients. I think that's probably going to be the biggest turnaround for the next couple years is the shift from mostly in labs to out of lab studies.

Dr. Gould: On that note. This is a half hour show, because as exciting as this is I wanted to limit to that. What I do want to just briefly talk about is in my office we are using the Aries take home sleep study, and I was really impressed by just the ease of use. We get this diagnosis. The sleep study goes to a sleep doctor who does the real diagnosis. As a dentist I can only identify and treat. I can't diagnose, which is perfectly fine with me. We talked about what I'm doing in my practice, and the things that have kept people away from treating it is I'm really working in the trenches here. I'm trying to get a feeling for what's going to change people's attitudes.

I think that for me to announce to the world everybody should get tested for sleep apnea is of no value, but the issue that we have is that with my patients they trust me. I've been here for 15 years. When they see what I'm going through I'm telling an honest story. I'm not trying to sell anyone anything. This is a very major issue, and I really hope that I can help you and myself to get this message out, because I think about the unnecessary pain that I went through because of my problems, and I think about all the people that we could really help to just avoid medication and torture and pain and all this stuff. I'm really excited. I would love to have you back in a future show to get more specific, but I want to let you go, because I know it's getting late on the East Coast. I really want to thank you so much for your time. I really appreciated you coming on my show.

Dr. Park: That's for having me. It was great to be here.

Dr. Gould: Thank you very much, and we'll speak to you soon. Have a great night. So we're at the end of our half hour. I've gone a bit over, but Dr. Park what I've gone through, what I've realized, what I've seen is so shocking, but he saw all this a couple years ago. What an interesting guy to put the pieces together and not have any kind of issue with wanting to work with dentists, because we're the ones who are in control of that whole area. I'm going to wrap things up here.

Next week I have an equally and probably a little more scary topic. I'm calling the segment All About the D. D stands for Vitamin D. I want to end this show by saying you do not want to miss the next episode, because I'm going to tell you some earthshattering things about Vitamin D, and Vitamin D is not a vitamin. It's a hormone. It looks like cholesterol or testosterone, and you can buy it over the counter. More interestingly, you can get it from the sun. I want to leave it at that.

I want to say thank you to everybody for listening. I can't wait for you to hear next week's podcast. Thank you so much for listening. Follow us at Modern American Dentistry on Facebook or our website at ModernAmericanDentistry.com. Thank you to my producer, Maria DiGiovanni. You're the best. Everybody, get your smile on. We'll see you soon.

GYSO – Eps. 6 Ivor Cummins Vitamin D

Dr. Gould: Everybody, hello out there and welcome to my international listening audience. This is Get Your Smile On, and I am Dr. Joel Gould, your wellness dentist, broadcasting live from beautiful Manhattan Beach, California in the offices of Modern American Dentistry. Tonight, as your wellness dentist, I've got an incredibly interesting story about something that you've heard about, a little something called Vitamin D. Today I am calling m show Vitamin D for Dummies. The reason is that Vitamin D is not a vitamin. When I got into the whole idea of wellness dentistry I didn't really know that I'd be getting interested in nutrition and vitamins.

My whole foray into this whole industry of wellness is something that has been really exciting for me, and after 25 years of the practice of dentistry, not that I find teeth boring, but I really like the idea, and always have, of treating a whole person as a whole person. The most important part of that is getting to know who that person is and learning about what their life is like and how we can make them feel happy and more comfortable. We've talked about a lot of different topics. Vitamin D, when I was in dental school we learned about how important Vitamin D was for healthy teeth and bones. I don't really remember learning a lot more about it than that.

Since I have gotten into the understanding that Vitamin D is not a vitamin, it is a hormone, it has really gotten my interest up, and the more I looked into this the more fascinated I was by what's really going on in the medical industry and the lack of understanding and information of what Vitamin D is. When you need to get your Vitamin D checked you have to have a blood test. It takes a few days.

There's different methods that they can test, but we're going to talk tonight to one of the most interesting speakers on the subject of Vitamin D, and we're just about to bring him on the phone. I actually want to say that I'm really excited about this episode. We're doing this a little later today. This is 10:00PM west coast time, because my guest is calling in from Ireland, and it is 6:00AM there. We want to thank him for getting up a little bit early. Today we're going to cover the really interesting things that you don't know about Vitamin D.

What I find interesting is I ask people, "Have you had your Vitamin D checked?" Everyone says, "I take supplements. I'm good." The most interesting part about that is people just being so dismissive about the idea that they could know that they're getting the right amount of Vitamin D. What we're going to talk about is the mistakes that Vitamin D has sort of had through history, and also the idea that the FDA, their recommendations for Vitamin D is 800 international units. We're going to talk about Vitamin D doses and international units. The reason we're going to do that is because the FDA and a lot of different medical professionals really haven't had the idea of how much you need and how do we regulate this?

I'm going to go ahead and bring on my guest tonight. I want to welcome Ivor Cummins to my show. Ivor, are you there?

Ivor: Hi there, Joel. Here I am.

Dr. Gould: How are you doing? We've got 10:00PM on the west coast, and I guess the sun's coming up in Ireland?

Ivor: It is indeed.

Dr. Gould: I want to thank you for arranging this to be with me on the show. I'm really excited. I know that you're a very technical speaker, and I've watched your presentations. They're medically very fascinating, but today with my show I'm focusing on sort of a broader audience that maybe isn't as well versed in the medical side. I sort of want to focus on a lot about how you came to be this sort of Vitamin D expert. I'd like my viewers to know your background. Tell us about yourself.

Ivor: Right, Joel. I'm a biochemical engineer originally. I'm at work for nearly 30 years now, mainly focusing on complex problem solving in the engineering sphere. I've really specialized in leading teams to solve complex problems, follow the right methodology, and obviously this turned out very useful when I got into the medical world a couple of years back, when I had my own health issues. I was able to research hundreds of papers. I understand the statistics. I understand the biochemistry. At one point, I came across D quite early, so I was studying metabolic syndrome, atherosclerosis, heart disease, and metabolism and carbohydrate and fat, which is kind of getting to be a big deal now, the low carbohydrate movement. Inevitably I came across Vitamin D, because it's profoundly connected to all of that and to so many things, as you've mentioned yourself.

Dr. Gould: Great. Because this is a half hour radio show I want to get right to your information, but there's lots of different connected topics that are related to everything that you just said. I want you to know that these are topics that I really am going to be covering in my future shows, because like you I've had some health issues that are related to the things that I'm getting interested in discussing. This is a very broad topic, and I've really asked you some difficult questions here, how to sort of summarize how this works in Vitamin D. I'm going to let you do your thing. We talked about humans and evolutions and all that, and I guess give me your best elevator pitch for how Vitamin D came up in the world. I don't know if they use that expression in Ireland, but that's pretty typical out here in Los Angeles.

Ivor: I work in the corporate world, so we got that phrase. I'll try and simplify. Basically, in terms of human evolution there's lots of different views, but I'll go with the primary one. Several hundred million years ago we left the seas, and in the sea vertebrates, animals with backbones, access calcium all around them, whereas when we moved onto the land you needed to get calcium through food and other forms and absorb it. So Vitamin D became a critical part of that. It enables the extraction of calcium and the absorption into the body to make bones and many other things. So very early on in our evolution Vitamin D became a very important part of our physiology. As a result, I believe it became importantly connected to many other control systems in the body, because it came so early.

Then for human evolution around 20,000 years ago, maybe 30,000, we migrated northwards, away from the high ultraviolet light environment of the equator, and that's where it's believed our skin coloration became increasingly white, and one of the key reasons was to access Vitamin D from UV sunlight energy, because there's so much less UV as you move northwards from the equator. Really in America, Northern Europe you've got a few months of the year where mainly in the midday period when the sun is directly overhead you access a lot of UV for Vitamin D production. Because it's so important for the body, it's believed that our skin lightened in order to access a lot more in environments where there was a lot less UV.

They have done studies linking human skin color from indigenous local populations from all over the world linking it to the available ultraviolet light and seeing very powerful correlations. So the human skin color basically tracks with UV availability, thus ensuring that you'll get plenty of Vitamin D production all around the world. That's kind of really a snapshot of how we've evolved to access this critical component.

Dr. Gould: I know that a lot of people may not know, or I think most people do understand that Vitamin D, the precursor to the active form is synthesized on our skin by sun exposure. Aside from that, where else would people get Vitamin D if they weren't getting their sun exposure?

Ivor: If you're not getting the sun exposure, and it's been hypothesized that the Inuit who are very far north with poor sun they have access to a lot of fatty fish. So you can get Vitamin D from organ meats, fatty fish, and a lot of foods that, to be quite honest, we don't eat a whole lot any more. So not only does the modern population, are we sun fearing, because of the dermatology scares, which are mostly invalid. We might get into that, but the population is also not eating Vitamin D rich food anymore. So cod liver oil, organ meats, fatty fish from cold water areas, they're the other sources, and, of course, to a certain extent in dairy products. Generally speaking the American population now, if you take an evolutionary level of hydroxy D in the blood that would have been the 40s, the average for the population is around 20, which is getting to the deficient level. Many people are below the deficient level.

Dr. Gould: I just want to clarify for our listeners. We're talking about a number like 20 or 40, and that's nanograms per microliter. That's how that is tested in the body. It's a standardized test.

Ivor: That's the standardized test. There are other units, but the US units nanograms per mL are probably the best ones. We won't confuse people with the other unit sys-tems. An evolutionary level of this component in the body created from the Vitamin D itself would be in the 40s, possibly in the 50s for women, but everyone is pretty much way below that now.

Dr. Gould: That's something that's really more coming to light these days, which is great, but when I discuss this with my patients a lot of times everyone's very quick to say, "I drink lots of milk, or I take a multivitamin." Having you on the show, I wanted to make sure that everyone understands from an expert point of view it doesn't really matter what you think you're getting. It's really about the level in your blood. When you take a vitamin it's different than when you have a hormone, so we're looking at a range aren't we? We want to be at a certain range, and that range would sort of change if you tested yourself every day. It wouldn't be the same. It would be a little bit variable.

Ivor: Yeah. There would be variability in the test, but gener-ally it's not a bad test, even if you take a one off read-ing. They've found that over time it doesn't change too much for people who have consistent behavior. The best range that I can come to to advise people is around 40-50 would be the range. There are some researchers who believe you should be higher. I'm not sure there's evidence to really back that up, and then the govern-ment, of course, seems to be happy with levels around in the 20s, which I would say the evidence would sug-gest is too low. 40-50 would be a good range, and the beauty is you can get this simple test, and then over a period of three to six months you can access sunlight, take supplements, and then get a test six months later and just verify that you're generally on the right track.

Dr. Gould: Before we talk about what happens when you don't have enough Vitamin D I want to talk about Vitamin D toxicity. How much Vitamin D would somebody have to take to feel a toxic effect?

Ivor:

That's a great question. The best data, and I've researched a lot, that I can come to if you take over 30,000 international units a day of supplements you're entering the area where you could go too high in Vitamin D. So to give a reference for people, if you go out in healthy sunlight with a lot of your body exposed, and maybe you become slightly pink, you will generate around 20,000 units in that day. Nature has provided us with the system through our skin that's able to produce 20,000 units in maybe half an hour or an hour. That'll give you an idea of what's natural to produce in a day.

The current guidelines say 800, but to be honest 4,000 or 5,000 a day has no chance of toxicity, and it's probably what you'll need if you're not accessing sunlight in order to get your blood levels up to good evolutionary levels. Let's say up to 10,000 a day is certainly not toxic.

Dr. Gould:

10,000 a day, people who are taking supplements, that would definitely be a lot. Much more interesting to my listeners, and really when I was listening to your presentation you talk about something called a smile curve. The smile curve should actually be a frown curve, shouldn't it?

Ivor:

Yeah. They're pretty impressive. The smile curve just shows that the incidence of many diseases get higher as you move away from the equator. There is an element that people away from the equator in more advanced societies they obviously eat more bad food and all that kind of stuff, but it's a very strong relationship where when you move from the equator you've less availability of ultraviolet light, and you tend to produce a lot less

Vitamin D, particularly during the winter. Many diseases become worse in those areas, multiple sclerosis, diabetes, obesity, and heart disease. If people wanted to follow this up there's a book called *Cholesterol and the Sun* by Dr. David Grimes available on Amazon, etc. It really goes into a lot of what we're talking today for the layperson.

They've even seen that the patterns, if you take France, the incidence of multiple sclerosis doesn't just follow the north to south, like the smile curve, it actually follows the weather patterns and where there is less cloud cover and where there is more sun availability. UV availability tracks with many diseases, and it's believed to be through the Vitamin D effect.

Dr. Gould: I just want to clarify. When we talk about what a smile curve is, this is sort of more for a scientist who likes to plot things onto a graph. If I got this straight, and if I'm explaining this properly, it is if you plot the diseases that we talked about, and it's pretty much almost every disease, when you plot this on a graph, and you do it in relation to your distance away from the equator when you look at that graph it makes sort of a smile shape along the X and Y axis, for anybody who still remembers that from their junior high or algebra or geometry.

This seems to be something that everybody should know about. This isn't some groundbreaking discovery. These are scientists have taken just general data, and they've plotted it on a graph. When did people start to know or see that there was this correlation between poor health and less availability of sunlight?

Ivor: Yeah, Joel, I'd say decades ago really it's known, but I think the general established orthodox kind of medical community, as you said, there's not a lot of awareness. So although in scientific circles there's an awareness, it's not generally publicized a lot. I'm not sure why exactly. There are very strong correlations. Some would argue that they're only correlations, and that can't prove cause. I guess that's true to an extent, but because the correlations or associations are so strong in those curves you really have to assume there's something going on there. Interestingly, if you go from north to south even within countries you see a shift in the disease. It's not just across the world. It's also within countries and across Europe from north to south you see the same relationship. It's very powerful, and it's kind of consistent wherever you go. It's very strong.

The important thing is that there are also the mechanisms. If something like that correlates or tracks it may not prove cause, but for Vitamin D there is so much research showing how it can affect those diseases that if you put everything together it's quite powerful.

Dr. Gould: Being sort of medically aware and having almost 30 years in it was really shocked. I thought I had seen most of the mysteries of life exposed, but to see this was, hopefully my listeners are beginning to understand that this is really kind of a shocking revelation that all of modern medicine, and especially in a place like California where health and wellness is so highly valued, this is literally really still just not known. I had a patient in today or yesterday who is a medical doctor, and we talked a little bit about it. He said he was very big on D, but we talked about it. He had absolutely no training. There was really just no information out there, and if medical doctors don't know then certainly the general public isn't going to know.

As we get towards the end of this I want to talk to you about what you're now working on, but I want to still focus on the Vitamin D, just because I know that you're sort of past this, and this passé. You've talking about this without the recognition that it deserves. I want to put a more common sense version of this for my listeners so they can understand why a chronic Vitamin D deficiency in America, how would that show up? We discussed back and forth about the idea of hibernation and winter and summer. I know that it's not super technical to talk about this, but I think that it would really give our listeners an understanding if we could maybe discuss about the move north of the border and what happens in spring with animals, mammals versus winter. How would you sort of explain that to the average person who's not completely aware of the whole Vitamin D story?

Ivor: The seasonal shift there's a lot of different theories. Again, diseases track seasonally. When many diseases, including tuberculosis back in the day and heart disease, to be honest too many to mention, the incidence or the amount of them increases when people are at their low Vitamin D level. Low Vitamin D again is associated with excessive disease rates, based on seasonal shifts. You can store Vitamin D, so if you access plenty in the summer and you can store the Vitamin in your fat, and it can kind of carry you through the winter. There are strong beliefs emerging that maintaining a steady D intake during the whole year has a lot of benefits. A lot of studies around that, and the best advice would be to keep your D level pretty consistent throughout.

Dr. Gould: Right. It makes perfect sense once you sort of become aware of this. One of the things that was also interesting to me is the idea that having an optimal level of Vitamin D would allow your intestinal flora, or the bacteria in your intestines, to make different types of chemical products, like B vitamins. Was that something that you were really looking into, or is that not the focus of what you were considering?

Ivor:

The whole gut health thing is really important. More of my expertise in that front would be around carbohydrate, that excess of carbohydrate and fructose and pretty much give you the wrong gut macrobiota, but Vitamin D does partake in that also, but it's not something I'd have gone so deep into, more the mechanisms connecting to disease. Vitamin D has a lot of mechanisms in the body that really mimic what some drugs attempt to do.

Just to your earlier question about the medical field, I think doctors are trained mainly in pharmaceutical intervention, recognize the disease, and then give it the right drug. I think if D is at a good level it has the effect that a lot of drugs would have. It enables processes to run much better, and you would not have as much need for the drug or treatment side. I think the medical profession really is educated not in nutrition or in the criticality of these vitamins, but more in identifying the problem and then applying the pharmaceutical.

Dr. Gould:

Right. That is welcome to America. What's funny about me is that as a wellness dentist, being in California, I'm also Canadian. The Canadian healthcare system is very different than the US healthcare system, and having lived in both countries I really see the differences. Although in Canada we do still have the same push to treat things with medications.

I wanted to talk just a little bit about the cancer connection here in two different ways. One is the idea that sun exposure causes cancer, and then the other is the Vitamin D connection with regard to people's DNA. I think those are two kind of really shocking facts that were brought to light when I heard you speak. Back to the elevator pitch, what's your best elevator pitch on how cancer, DNA, and sun exposure fit together?

Ivor:

Cancer's a really interesting one. I think, if I try and simplify it, there's been an idea for many decades now that the sun causes cancer. Keep out of the sun. Less the better. Which is obviously an absurd idea. We evolved with the sun. It creates D. It creates nitrous oxide. It expands your blood vessels. There's a huge amount of beneficial effects from the sun. We evolved with it. This idea for a few decades has been it causes cancer. People might not be aware, there's only around 2,000 deaths a year from the classic simple skin cancers. They're very common, but there's a very low mortality rate. You can treat them relatively easily.

However, there's around 8,000 or 9,000 deaths a year from melanoma, which is the really nasty skin cancer. The thing about melanoma is most good studies show that getting more sun exposure means you'll have a lower rate of melanoma. The reason is that healthy sun exposure keeps your Vitamin D high, and your skin protects itself by releasing melanin and by tanning. So the irony is that more healthy sun exposure without burning actually links to lower rates of the serious skin cancer, the one with the high mortality. Unfortunately, the whole dermatology world for the last 40 years has nonstop driven this idea that sun causes cancer.

Even a lot of sunblocks nowadays, they actually block the UVB, which creates Vitamin D, and they allow through the UVA. The UVA, there's a lot more UVA in the sun's energy, and it's the UVA in many studies that links more closely to cancer generation. The funny thing is people with sunblocks were losing their Vitamin D, losing the benefits of UVB, while the sunblock was allowing through the UVA, which is more closely linked to cancer generation, the melanoma. The whole sun and cancer thing has been, I think, completely mixed up, and as a result people are staying away from healthy sun, evolutionary sun, and they're losing out on all the benefits. It's pretty mixed up.

Dr. Gould: It's one of those things that when you start to come up against the American medical community, and that's such a strong belief they have that any sun exposure is dangerous. What I like about the whole issue is that I think about the pharmacy companies that are going to lose money if people were to have their optimum Vitamin D level, a lot of medication use would go down, but I think those people should probably reinvest in the vacation and safe sun exposure industry. I think we could probably have a lot more fun with resorts where you go for your Vitamin D than going to a hospital and getting some chemicals that are just basically putting a Band-Aid on what's a larger issue. It's pretty incredible. Thank you so much for how articulate you are in getting that message across. It's really great to hear.

Before we get to the end of the show, is there anything about Vitamin D in all your work and studies that really struck you that you want to sort of leave my listeners with so that they can understand a little bit more about this crazy topic?

Ivor: Yeah. Elevator pitch on that one. I guess to keep in mind that you make 20,000 units a day easily in the healthy sun exposure without burning, so that should give people an idea of what nature pretty much intended. Why would the body create 20,000 units in a day of something unless it had a reason? Therefore taking a few thousand units a day while tracking your blood with a test occasionally can get you into that 40+ evolutionary range. D level is connected to so many diseases. It's kind of bizarre in a sense, but it also, without getting into detail here, has detailed technical mechanisms as to why it would connect to those diseases. It's not really a mystery.

Without going into detail, there are many, D actually enables you to go into your DNA, your very DNA, to unwind it and create molecules that help create enzymes to deal with infections and deal with other problems. I think you mentioned earlier, Joel, if people realized their DNA is not just kind of sitting there, or enables you to procreate. Your DNA is accessed all the time in your 40 trillion cells, and it is unwound, the two strands, and you encode off proteins and enzymes, depending on what your body needs. It's a living library, and Vitamin D is intimately connected into accessing that library properly to access the code of our evolution for helping us with health problems and running your system.

It's really profound, and everyone should be around the evolutionary level, ideally, but over probably three quarters or more are below the evolutionary level we would have had as humans thousands of years ago.

Dr. Gould: It's just incredible. I know in America, that's what hear around the world, but is this known in a lot of other countries, or is it better known in other places and most Americans are not knowing or ignoring it?

Ivor: It's a worldwide problem, Joel, because a lot of the worldwide health community has kind of followed the US lead and the guidelines. It's a worldwide problem. In the UK now rickets is actually making a return, so from the industrial revolution in the 1800s we had children with malformed bones from lack of sun exposure. It's actually coming back in the UK now after 20 or 30 years of bad science, I would say.

Dr. Gould: That's absolutely unbelievable. First of all, I just want to thank you for going back into the Vitamin D world, but now I want to talk to you about what you're working on now. I was following on your website, which we're going to give to our listeners at the end here. It's a little different focus. Maybe not another elevator pitch, but this is something that you're really into. I'd love you to explain to me and to my listeners what it is that you're working on.

Ivor: Okay. Really what I've been working on the past while, I'm doing a book, and I'm funded by a philanthropist. It's to explain a couple of things. One is the calcium scan of the heart, the CT scan, which is very inexpensive, and it really tells you if you have heart disease in your arteries like no other technology. You get a CAC score, and that will basically show you. You can have someone who is high risk, and they can get a scan and find out that they have zero calcium in their arteries, and they're actually in good shape, or likewise you could appear to be healthy and slim, like my sponsor, and find out that your arteries are in terrible shape, and you've got advanced heart disease. It's to get that message out there about this CT scan of the heart.

Then also to explain how to avoid heart disease. A lot of that has to do with the hormone insulin, and our modern population is suffering massively from high insulin, metabolic syndrome, middle obesity, and heart disease. A lot that relates to excessive carbohydrates driving up your insulin levels. I can't go into detail here. That's what the book's about.

Dr. Gould: As I read on your website, and I was sort of wondering, we have all these processed carbohydrates and back 30,000 years ago did our ancestors eat any carbohydrates that we would consider very healthy that we want to include in our diets?

Ivor: Yeah. They would have seasonally had access in the

Northern Hemisphere to fruits. They would have been lower sugar fruits though, and they would have only got them at certain times in the year, whereas now everyone's gorging on high sugar fruits all year around. That's a problem. They also would have accessed tubers and underground tubers, but they would have been eating a lot of above ground vegetables, which are low in sugar and glucose. So they would have been eating carbohydrates, but far healthier than what we eat today.

Once you process them you take away a lot of the goodness. You're left with pure glucose sugar, and that sends your insulin crazy. It's a massive problem nowadays where people's insulin levels are way above where they should be, and that promotes fat storage. It stops you healthily burning your own fat, and it basically drives a whole host of diseases. Insulin, I think, in the next decade is going to be the big story. They've underestimated the damage from high insulin for 50, 60 years, at least.

Dr. Gould: Before we close the show, this is all similar topic is that we have the entire American medical industry sort of running in a completely different direction than what you have been looking into. Do you see any hope? Are there messages getting out there? Do you see a little bit of a turn of the tide for America and for how we're viewing our health?

Ivor: I think it's beginning, Joel. The 2016 dietary guidelines, a preview has been sent out, and they are dropping dietary cholesterol from the guidelines. It's no longer of concern. I think this was known decades ago around the world. They're also beginning to pull away from recommending low fat diets, which quite frankly have been a disaster and have been a large part of the diabetes and obesity epidemic, pushing higher carb, and they're realizing that now. Even the official authorities that have not moved for 20, 30 years, even though the scientific evidence shows they should have, are beginning to move.

I was just in South Africa in February, and the world's first low carbohydrate summit was on, and I was part of that. We had 20 experts from all around the world, doctors, PhDs, specialists, speaking for four days on the perils of carbohydrate. It was a huge event, and people can look it up on the web. I think the world is beginning to realize, with the internet, with access to scientific papers like I was able to get through the internet, smart people around the world are beginning to realize they really mixed things up 50 years ago or 40 years ago when they pushed high carb guidelines. All that I think in the next 10 years is going to completely shift.

Dr. Gould: I really hope so. Part of me doing this show is to actually help to push things in that direction. Some of my other shows that I have and will have covered are really a lot of preventive care talk. In dentistry preventive care saves thousands of dollars and pain and time in the chair, just the same way that preventive care of your body by eating and getting the right amount of safe sun exposure can really decrease a lot of people's pain, agony, and suffering.

I want to let everybody know how they can get a hold of you. If you want to give out your website address, go ahead.

Ivor: Thanks, Joel. It's www.thefatemperor.com.

Dr. Gould: I love it. That's a great name. I'd love to have you on a later show to speak about this, and I'd love to even know how you came up with that name. That sounds pretty incredible. I love the idea also that eating relatively healthy meat and cheese is back on the diet, because they're pretty great.

Ivor: Yeah, and there's no better way to protect your teeth than to back off on that carbohydrate.

Dr. Gould: Definitely. Hold on, I've got to have some business. No. I'm in the promotion of health here, and there's no secret about how to get rid of tooth decay. It's funny how it all fits together.

I want to thank you so much for coming on my show. I really appreciate it. You are my first international guest, and I'd love to have you on the show again. Thank you.

Ivor: For sure. Thanks a lot. It's been a pleasure.

Dr. Gould: Great. Hopefully we'll speak to you soon. All right, everybody. I hope that if you're listening live that kind of shocked you, because, like I said, when I learned about this I was really blown away. There's so many interesting topics that this opens up, health and wellness and wellness dentistry, absolutely. Vitamin D is a very interesting issue, and in future episodes I want to talk about the link between Vitamin D and sleep, sleep apnea and sleep breathing disorders. I've got some incredible guests who can maybe take us down that road.

That's it for tonight. I want to thank all of you for listening. I want to thank my incredible producer, and happy birthday, Maria DiGiovanni. You're the best. Until next time, get your smile on. I look forward to seeing you. Follow us on Twitter and Facebook, Modern American Dentistry, and fairly soon hopefully we'll have these podcasts posted on iTunes. Thank you for listening, and we'll see you next week.

GYSO – Eps. 7 Dr. Mark Cruz Sleep Apnea

Dr. Gould: Hello, everybody out there. This is Get Your Smile On with me, Dr. Joel Gould, your wellness dentist. I am broadcasting live from beautiful Manhattan Beach, California. We have an incredibly exciting show tonight, and we have our guest who's going to be Dr. Mark Cruz, and we'll be getting to him shortly. As per usual, we're talking about wellness dentistry. In the past shows I've mentioned, made sort of an admission, that I found that I have something called sleep apnea.

Tonight we're going to actually talk about the larger group of conditions that we're calling sleep disordered breathing. What that really means is when you are trying to get your good night's sleep there is some issue with your airway that is preventing you from getting that good night's sleep. If we think back to the old days and our grandparents and what used to be going on back in the day, there is nothing better than a good night's sleep. These days it seems that we have a lot of medications, that's for sure, but what I want to talk about is the idea that having a good night's sleep is critical to who we are as people. It is only in sleep, and it is only in the deeper stages of sleep, that our bodies can truly heal themselves.

Everyone's heard of REM sleep, rapid eye movement. That's the point in our sleep cycle where our whole body becomes paralyzed. When our bodies become paralyzed, our airway also can become paralyzed. What sleep disordered breathing is is a list of different conditions that happen to people while they're sleeping, and particularly in the deep stages of sleep. Why is this so serious? We've talked about sleep apnea before and how deadly it can be, and we're going to talk about it more.

We're going to break it down, but what's really crazy about sleep apnea is that it prevents you from getting quality sleep.

We all have a whole genetic profile that we're programed to have, and our bodies are these incredible machines that have hormones and chemical mediators that will repair our bodies and keep us functioning well. When we are not getting the right amount of sleep, and it's not 8 hours. Maybe for some people it is 8 hours, but if you're not getting at least 5 good hours of sleep then you're very sleep deficient. That's a major issue. If you're sleep deficient your whole life is going to be affected.

How do you feel when you wake up and you haven't had a good night's sleep? Pretty terrible. How would you feel if you woke up not having a good night's sleep over and over and over again? After a certain point in time that would be normal, and so the admission I made by having sleep apnea is that I really didn't know that I was having problems. I was, and now that I've become more educated on this topic I really see all the signs that I've been missing.

What I want to go over real quickly here, before I bring my guest on, is why is a dentist even talking about sleep and sleep disorders? The answer's very obvious. Besides the fact that all day long I see people, and I look right down their airways with the bright lights, very different than most doctors. I have a completely different perspective about what someone's airway looks like. In addition to that, the very clear signs of sleep disordered breathing are bruxism, grinding of your teeth. I am a great dentist when it comes to making brux guards. I made one for myself. I made many for myself. They work really well. What that brux guard or grinding guard does is it's just masking the true issue that I have, and that is sleep disordered breathing and sleep apnea.

Not everybody has sleep apnea, but a lot of people do. There's something that's out there that's a little different called UARS, upper airway resistance syndrome. We've mentioned this before, and we're going to talk about it more. This is the petite female version of sleep apnea. Everyone thinks sleep apnea is a larger man with a big neck, and the truth is that sleep apnea can affect anyone and everyone. There's a huge genetic component to it, and it's very important that the symptoms and signs are seen and noticed, because early intervention will lead to a much easier treatment. The likelihood of someone needing to go on a more serious treatment such as a C-PAP machine would be reduced.

We are doing a treatment called a mandibular advancement device. I'm calling it a mandibular adjustment device, because we adjust how you have your mandible to open your airway. When it comes to UARS, the problem is that people who are having a hard time with their sleep, nobody thinks they have sleep apnea, because they shouldn't. The reality is this is something that's going on all around us.

Today we're going to be talking to my guest, who is a dentist in Orange County, and he has been dealing with this for a lot longer than I have. We're going to get all of his insights. Before we do that, I just want to go to a quick commercial break, and then we're going to be bringing our guest on, Dr. Mark Cruz. I'll be right back.

All right, everybody, welcome back. Tonight my guest is Dr. Mark Cruz. Dr. Cruz, are you there?

Dr. Cruz: I am here, Joel. How are you? Can you hear me?

Dr. Gould: Fantastic. I can hear you just great. Thank you so much for calling in. How's it going tonight?

Dr. Cruz: It's going fantastic. Thank you for asking.

Dr. Gould: Tonight we have so many things that I want to get to, but I want you just to tell my listeners who you are and what's been going on in your dental practice. Why don't you go ahead and introduce yourself?

Dr. Cruz: My name is Mark Cruz. I've been practicing since 1986 down in south Orange County, California. Our paths, Joel, as you know, our paths crossed as a result of Steven Park, who wrote the book *Sleep Interrupted*. He has actually been a speaker in my mini residencies going up to a number of individuals that speak on this very complex topic, which is not necessarily about sleep, more about airway functioning, dysfunction. Although often times we focus on sleep, disturbed sleep, just being a symptom rather than the cause. It's a symptom of a bigger problem, which is airway dysfunction, which is a common problem in our species, homosapiens, the last 500 or so years. It's a worldwide problem. I've been focusing more and more the last 8-10 years in my practice, and yet it is completely germane to what we do as dentists in restorative dentistry. Did that answer your question?

Dr. Gould: Absolutely. I guess I'll just clarify that we came in contact through Dr. Steven Park, and you've actually put together a group of medical professionals, including doctors and dentists and other allied healthcare professionals, because this is an issue that affects all of us, and someone you know. You were doing a mini residency, so for our conversation this is because this is not a well-known issue, all of this sleep disordered breathing and issues with airway.

Before we talk about how you got your group together, I want to get into how you came on to this topic. As a good dentist, we're taught a lot in dental school, and we gain a lot of experience out there in the real world. Each dentist has their own personality, and their practice may move towards one direction or another, orthodontics or root canals. What got you into the whole idea of sleep disordered breathing and airway?

Dr. Cruz: Pretty much from the outset I was always focused on comprehensive global treatment with the emphasis on diagnosis versus just drilling and filling or veneers or crowns or whatever. I always pursued a continuation in my education in treating what is known as gnathology and occlusion.

Dr. Gould: I wanted to interrupt, so you're saying gnathology and occlusion. For our listeners, I know you're so used to talking to dental professionals. Gnathology starts with a G. This is about how people's teeth come together and how they chew and how they function. I'll let you continue.

Dr. Cruz: Right. Exactly. I was just going to explain that. Those are fancy words for how the upper and the lower jaw function together with the temporomandibular joint and the teeth being just a part of a complex system. I use the fancy terms somatognathic system that describes the muscles, the bones, the joints, the ligaments, the tendons, the suspensory muscles of the neck that allow us to eat, speak, breathe. This is really what we deal with in dentistry, although we may choose to focus on one part of it like the teeth or the gums or the temporomandibular joints or the muscles. They don't work by themselves. They work in a synergy with each other, and in fact are part of the whole body in the way the entire body works.

That's mostly what I would work on, complex full mouth rehabilitations. People would come in with problems, often times to fix problems that were created many times by the dentist where unwittingly they would take care of a tooth that was hurting without really asking the question, why was the tooth hurting? Maybe it was because there was night grinding, as an example, what we call sleep bruxism. In more recent years coming out of the medical literature, specifically sleep medicine, we're starting to understand more that nocturnal bruxism and grinding, and even diurnal clenching, are related to airway dysfunction or sleep disordered breathing as part of an arousal response to maintain our proper breathing and airway function.

I started more and more focusing on dealing with the underlying problem versus the symptom. Traditionally we go ahead and say, "You're grinding. Let's make a night guard." The problem is although it mitigates the effect of the clenching and the grinding on the teeth, often times it makes the airway problem worse. That's a kind of synopsis.

Dr. Gould: Sure. The regular listeners on my show will know that I have defined what wellness dentistry is, and really I've defined it fairly clearly that we can't separate the teeth and the mouth. It's a part of the whole body. As dentists we're doctors of the mouth and all the associated structures, so it was really nice to hear you sort of summarize that. We talked that I've been a good boy giving my patients brux guards or grinding guards when I see signs of wear, and you're absolutely true that the biggest issue when it comes to sleep disordered breathing is that it isn't just dentists. It's the medical professionals, medical field in general.

We're treating a lot of the symptoms, and that's why I think that this makes sense that you were looking at the whole body. It makes perfect sense that you would have gotten into this. As far as I'm concerned this is quite a ways back, so you're definitely one of the leaders, or one of the most forward thinking people when it comes to this. In your practice did you come across this on a regular basis then you investigated, or you just said there's more to this and I want to investigate? What brought you to this position? How did you get interested in it?

Dr. Cruz:　In taking the philosophical approach that I just described I always questioned and always asked why versus just how do we do this? I think it led me to that. Also having somewhat of an accident career being at UCLA and teaching and being on faculty and being in the faculty group practice for 10 years or so. Doing research. I guess it created a mindset to critically think about these things and ask why? What is the evidence to support what we're doing? What I found often times is it was butting up against dogma that I was taught that didn't fit well with me. The reasons why I was told that things happen just didn't make sense. So that's why I started going outside of the discipline of dentistry per say and started looking in other areas.

The problem is in healthcare in general in the United States specifically, to some extent in Canada, but less so, is that we focus on managing disease instead of making people well. We have gotten very good at managing disease symptoms. The American public want a quick easy fix. They want that pill. They want that device. They want that surgery. Then they're in, they're out, and they're done. Unfortunately that's not really the way things work with our bodies.

Dr. Gould:　You touched on a lot of things there. Being Canadian myself, living half of my life in Canada and half of my life here, I'm really familiar with both medical systems. I still haven't quite figured out the US system yet, but being somebody who has been guilty, when I first started getting into sleep apnea, before I knew that I had this issue myself personally, it didn't make much sense to me what was going on. If people have this disorder why are more people not finding it out? I know now that just really no one's looking at it. People have an idea of what sleep apnea is, and they don't know that there's sleep disordered breathing that could be anyone and everywhere.

One of the things that I really like about the Canadian system in theory is that it's more based on science and research rather than drug companies trying to push their drugs. I don't want to blame anybody, because I think that we're all sort of guilty of just treating symptoms, especially as I see my bruxism patients as they come in day by day, and I have to tell them, "I've misdiagnosed you. There's something deeper going on here." In some cases.

What would you say, as for bruxism, because that's what we see so much in dentistry, what would you say the percentage of people who have obvious bruxism that is definitely related to sleep disordered breathing versus just what we would normally consider I'm under stress I grind my teeth? How do you think that breaks down?

Dr. Cruz: We actually spend quite a bit of time in that discussion. It's a hot topic. The evidence is mixed, and the problem with the evidence is the population that's looked at. First of all, let me just break it down. Obstructive sleep apnea is an end stage diagnosis. Another way of saying that is it's like let's look at cancer. Obstructive sleep apnea, when you have full blown obstructive sleep apnea, moderate to severe, that's like saying you've got Stage IV cancer or Stage III cancer. It's late stage. Our role really is to detect it before it becomes clinical, like carcinoma in situ or where you're at risk of developing cancer. So sleep disordered breathing is a spectrum where we're focusing just on the end stage. I would say obstructive sleep apnea is really just the tip of the iceberg of a major problem that is so pandemic worldwide.

Just think about this. Someone's who got obstructive sleep apnea, they're suffering from two types of big events. One's called an apnea, and one's called a hypopnea. An apnea is where your stop breathing for 10 seconds or more, and a hypopnea is where we have 30% of oxygen coming into the system or air coming into the system for 10 seconds or more. It's somewhat of an arbitrary cutoff for diagnosing a condition. Think about it. Physiologically the reason somebody stops breathing for 10 seconds or more while their sleeping is because something has gone wrong. There is damage in the central nervous system that says, if you stop breathing, no problem. It gets worse and worse.

Those individuals often times are not very symptomatic. If you actually talk to an obstructive sleep apnea patient they say, "It's no big deal. Might bother my spouse. I snore a little bit, but I'm fine. No problem." They're not even aware how much damage there is.

Dr. Gould: Mark, I want to interrupt you and say that I unfortunately was one of those people. I really didn't know that I had a problem, but in retrospect looking backwards everything that I have sort of come to know makes perfect sense. I feel a little embarrassed that I really should have recognized these symptoms, because as I'm seeing my patients a lot of them now that I mention this to some of them are saying, "I think maybe I might be having an issue." There's a lot of denial as well, because I know that people jump right to a C-PAP machine. They don't want to wear that gas mask forever.

I interrupted you. Sorry to stop you there. Go ahead. Go on.

Dr. Cruz: You're right. That's part of the problem. I've had patients say, "I don't care if I die. I'm not going to wear that mask." They don't understand that, first of all, there are many options to get the person out of a mask or not needing it to begin with. The point I'm trying to make, it's about early diagnosis. In fact, this can start as early as birth. We know that that is the case. Ron Harper from the UCLA brain research institute actually has done some studies as well as others, looking at children, premature babies or very young babies that can have what's called periodic breathing. It can start as early as the first year of life. It can actually cause brain damage that manifests and the snowball continues to build, if you will, and finally by the time it's caught it's already the individual's had this condition literally for decades.

A real important point I'd like to make. Individuals that are the most symptomatic are those individuals where it's earlier in the spectrum, and the reason for the awareness of symptoms and signs is because they're relatively healthy. Their autonomic nervous system is keeping them alive, keeping them breathing, which is the most important thing that we do from the moment that we're born to the day that we die, from one moment to the next. Not one hour to the next or one day to the next, but one moment to the next. Our entire physiologic systems are driven to protect that first and foremost, whether it's our metabolic system, our cardiovascular system, our brain function, our digestive function. That evidence is very clear. So many of the symptoms that an individual will report are related to that, yet those dots aren't connected, even by the primary care physician, the internist, the cardiologist.

That's the problem. We're looking at symptoms and not looking back at why is this occurring. An example, anxiety, depression, irritable bowel syndrome, chronic fatigue. Those all fall into the category of functional somatic syndromes that are functions of our airway dysfunction. I could on in more detail.

Dr. Gould: Okay. This is a half an hour show, and these are such interesting and important topics. From previous shows I have already confessed that myself personally I'm sort of the poster boy for this, because from a very early age I had problems. I was diagnosed with Crohn's disease, which is an autoimmune disease, but I also did not see an orthodontist until I was 13 years old. I was one of those kids that had the typical very retruded jaw, and I had a high narrow vaulted palate, and I had terrible allergies, so my nasal passages were completely blocked. I know looking back that it's kind of sad for me to think that it's taken us this long to figure this out, and I know that me being treated for my sleep apnea now I don't know what it's going to do for my Crohn's disease, but I do know that raising awareness on this incredibly huge topic, if I can spare one single child the childhood and medical issues that I have I'm willing to do anything to do that. That is sort of part of why I wanted to have you on the show, and why I really want to get the message out.

Wellness dentistry tends to come back to a lot of sleep apnea and sleep disordered breathing, but the reality is, and what I've come to learn and what most people are maybe just starting to figure out, is that this is everywhere and, again, I have a lot of patients they fill out their paperwork, they go to see a psychiatrist. The psychiatrist says, what's the problem? I'm anxious or depressed. Here's a prescription. There's no thought that this could be an underlying issue causing that. I'm here with you. I know that we spoke, and my job and my goal, because after a dentist of 25 years' experience just doing general dentistry, to me this is the most important topic in public health, medical care, that's global really.

I just wanted to make it clear to everybody that we're understanding this. The message is not getting out there as much as it should, but I think we're working on it. We've got a few minutes left before we close. I wanted to ask you. You have your regular patients who you see, do you have people who send people to see you?

Dr. Cruz: Yeah, more and more now. In my local community I literally interface with my patient's physicians in integrating their care on a daily basis. Those physicians, whether it's an internist, cardiology, primary care physician, pulmonologist, sleep physician, neurologist, psychiatrist, OB-GYN, literally.

Dr. Gould: Everyone.

Dr. Cruz: They will refer patients to me, because they're understanding we've shared patients together. They're actually connecting the dots themselves as well, and we actually now are collaborating in what we call the multidisciplinary wellness collaboration, where we actually do case reviews on a video conference on a regular basis looking at our patients, beyond just our individual specialties. It's continued to increase and normal people in the public are demanding wellness. The whole question, just like the whole question on ADHD. We now know that most ADHD is caused by fragmentation of sleep, and put them on drugs. What are those drugs? It's speed. Really the first thing we should be looking at with our kids is how they're sleeping.

Dr. Gould: You brought up a lot of great points, and I want to have the opportunity to have you back on my show again. It is a half hour show, because I don't want to keep people occupied. I want to thank you so much, and I would love to have you back on a more specific topic. I think you really helped my listening audience understand what kind of a major issue this is. I thank you so much for your time. I look forward to seeing you very soon.

Dr. Cruz: Sounds good. Take care, Joel.

Dr. Gould: Thanks, Mark. Bye. Okay, everybody, we're just about out of time, and I want to say thank you to my producer, Maria DiGiovanni. You're the best. You can find us on SoundCloud and soon to be on iTunes, and our website. You can find Mark Cruz at www.MarkACruzDDS.com. Look him up on Google. He's great if you're in Orange County and you have an issue. Give him a call. All right, everybody, thank you so much. I look forward to next week's show where I'll have some pretty fantastic mind-blowing exciting guests. Thank for listening to Get Your Smile On. Have a great night. Goodbye.

GYSO – Eps. 8
Dr. Dennis Goodman Magnesium

Dr. Gould: All right, everybody. Welcome to Get Your Smile On. This is Dr. Joel Gould, your wellness dentist, broadcasting live from beautiful Manhattan Beach, California. It's a beautiful sunny day here. It is 2:00PM, and we have a little different show today. We have adjusted our schedule to accommodate Dr. Dennis Goodman, an incredible cardiologist who we're going to bring on very shortly.

Today's topic is one of wellness, and everybody knows that I've been getting into sleep apnea, because I have it, discussing it and sleep disordered breathing. In my search and research for how to provide my patients with the highest level of care when it comes to sleep and what we do here in this office I came across the supplement of magnesium. In fact, we're going to call it magnificent magnesium, because this is an element that is absolutely spectacular. Magnesium was named after the Greek city of Magnesia, which was known for its fertile soil, which was really rich in magnesium. Magnesium is the eighth most abundant element on the earth, and the eleventh most abundant element in the body. Magnesium has been part of our cellular history since we evolved in the ocean and crawled up onto the shore.

Today Dr. Goodman, who is a board certified cardiologist from South Africa. He is also certified in internal medicine at Montefiore in, I believe, Pennsylvania. His book *Magnificent Magnesium*, just the cover alone tells you how important this is. It helps avoid heart attacks. It lowers blood pressure. It stops painful muscle cramps. It relieves nagging insomnia and increases calcium absorption. When I started to do my research into magnesium and why this would be so important I was brought back to my early high school days when we learned about energy and the Krebs Cycle.

Everybody knows about a crazy little thing called ATP, adenosine triphosphate. This is a chemical compound that is responsible for powering every single cellular function that you have in every one of the trillion cells you have in your body. Without adenosine triphosphate, or ATP, nothing works. The thing that people have either forgotten or, I guess I didn't know, this was already a long time ago for me, but magnesium is actually a very important part of the ATP complex.

In fact, without magnesium the ATP is not functional. So it would make sense that if you don't have enough magnesium you don't have any energy. This is something that is little known. We see all types of advertising for CoQ10 and this supplement and Vitamin C and EmergenC. This is one of the lesser known elements that we need, and it's critical to all of our bodily functions, and especially that of the heart. The heart is the most important muscle in the body. In fact, 25% of all deaths come from heart disease.

What I want to talk about today is a way that maybe western medicine hasn't focused on as closely as they should have, considering that we often wait until someone shows signs of cardiac problems, chest pains, high blood pressure. By the time these disease processes start to really affect us, things are actually pretty bad. Most of modern medicine goes in at the level where we're going to try and reduce your blood pressure. We are going to try and stabilize the way your heart is beating, or a lot of times we don't get to look at these details until after someone's already had a heart attack.

Today my guest is really the preeminent expert on

magnesium. He's also written three other books. His other book is *Thrill of Krill*. We'll have to ask him about that. Anybody who doesn't know what krill is, you can ask the great and mighty Google. He always knows. His more recent book that has just come out is called *K2, the Missing Nutrient for Heart and Bone Health*. This is actually one of the areas that I was most interested in, because as a dentist we look at calcium. We look at bone. We look at all types of things that are involved in the jaw and healing.

The Vitamin K2 is the missing link, or the missing piece, that I think that a lot of researchers don't really know what our issue is when it comes to having hardening in our arteries. When it comes to high blood pressure and stroke these are things that happen because our blood pressure gets to be too high, and why does that happen? All of our blood vessels are lined with cells that are called endothelial cells. These cells are very specific, and they line every single blood vessel in our entire body. It is these cells that take up calcium and give off calcium, depending on the right type of electrolytes we have and our diet, the amount of calcium we're eating, the amount of magnesium we have in our bodies. When we take extra calcium it doesn't necessarily go into our bones. We need a variety of cofactors of different cellular enzymes that all work together to metabolize calcium and take it out of the blood stream and put it into the bone where it can give you bone strength.

As you know, as we get older a lot of people end up being on calcium supplements because their bones are brittle. What we can do a little bit ahead of getting to the stage where our bones are brittle is we could consider the idea that there's only one way to get the calcium out of our arteries and into our bone, and that is with the right chemical mediators. Of course we will talk about magnesium, but Vitamin K2 is a little known vitamin, and it's one that you're going to probably hear a lot more about. I really look forward to bringing you all the latest and greatest on this particular vitamin.

We're still waiting for Dr. Goodman to come online here. I'm going to go on just a bit further about a few things here. We've been talking a lot about sleep apnea and different issues that people are having with their sleep. Magnesium is a very useful element when it comes to that. Magnesium is what we burn through when we're stressed, so when we're having a stressful day emotionally or physically we really metabolize a ton of magnesium. If we burn through all our magnesium, our body is going to start to react by having difficulty both with our heart pumping blood and also with us even just generally feeling like we have energy. It makes perfect sense that if we took the supplement we would be feeling a little more energized.

What is wrong with society today that we do not have enough magnesium in our diets? Magnesium was everywhere. It was in all the soil in all the farmlands in all the Western world. Over many years of farming the magnesium has been depleted from the soil. As a result, the foods that we eat are deficient in magnesium. In fact, there's a lot of statistics that show that almost every American is deficient on their magnesium. Since this is such an important element with regards to heart health, it's really incredible that the whole medical industry hasn't sort of taken a little closer look at something that's natural, something that we used to get from the garden, something we used to actually be in contact with as we walked in bare feet. Throughout our evolutionary journey we were in contact with this element. You can get it into your system by soaking your feet in Epson salts. It does cross over your cellular membranes.

You don't just get magnesium from taking it.

I kind of want to go back to a different time, maybe 10,000 years ago or 20,000 years ago or even 40,000 years ago, where we as the incredible organic animals that we are today evolved. We evolved under different conditions. We didn't wear shoes. We didn't have paved streets. We were in contact with the soil a lot more, and absorbing magnesium. Here we are, this incredibly evolved animal, really living in a beautiful gilded air-conditioned comfortable cage, shielding ourselves from dangerous rays of the sun, and preventing our bodies from touching the magnesium that's out there everywhere in the world. So when we go back to more basic diets, and we look at raw food diets and different diets that are rich in vegetables, we see that people who follow these diets have higher levels of magnesium, simply because of the way their diet is.

We're going to take a commercial break here in one second, and I'm going to go see if we can chase down Dr. Dennis Goodman. He is calling in from Manhattan, and I do believe that he's had a pretty busy day. We're going to go to a commercial break in just one second, and we'll hopefully come back with Dr. Dennis Goodman. Sorry to keep you all in such suspense. Let's hang on for one quick second for our commercial break.

All right, everybody, we are back live on the air, and we definitely have a little technical glitch here. We're still waiting—oh, we have him on. Dr. Goodman, are you there?

Dr. Goodman: Hello, Dr. Gould. How are you?

Dr. Gould: Please call me Joel. Thank you so much. Welcome to the show. Glad we got you.

Dr. Goodman: Thank you. Sorry there a little glitch getting through, but I hope I didn't keep you waiting.

Dr. Gould: You'll be able to hear when we post this on the website, but what's interesting is that I did read your book, and I read it cover to cover. It was a good thing, because I had to kind of wing a lot of the stuff that I wanted to ask you about. So hopefully I did your book some justice.

                  We can just jump right into it. I gave people a little bit of your background. Why don't you just tell us a little bit about yourself and where you're at right now?

Dr. Goodman: It goes back to many years ago I was born in South Africa, and I went to medical school at the University of Cape Town. It's associated with Groote Schuur Hospital where they did the first heart transplant by Christiaan Barnard in 1967. So I was very privileged to be there to train. Then I came to the United States, and I did my residency in Pittsburgh, and I did my cardiology fellowship at Baylor in Houston, where Dr. Michael Devecchi was another legend. I went to the cardiology program that was associated with his cardiac surgery program, and he did the first bypass surgery in 1955. I've been trained by these giants. I'm very lucky, because what happens is you get inspired, and then I decided to go to San Diego, and I was there for 20 years. I actually did invasive cardiology and was ultimately very involved Scripps. I was the Head of Cardiology at Scripps Memorial for many years.

                  I started to realize when I was putting stents in and opening up arteries when people were having heart attacks that I started to feel a bit like a fireman when you go to a house that's burning down. Sometimes you manage to stop the fire and save the house and save the people, and it's a little bit like that when you're trying to take care of people having a heart attack. Obviously you feel so good if you can really help somebody, and sometimes you can't, because it's too late. I really started to focus on where I think it's really at if we're going to make a real difference, and that is prevention and getting people to take responsibility for their health early on.

I know you know this, Joel, but 80% of chronic illnesses, like atherosclerosis, diabetes, obesity, many inflammatory conditions, arthritis, a lot of that stuff is reversible. If you start early enough, and the word really is preventable. 80% of these conditions are actually preventable. So then I started moving into the whole arena, and I've always been interested in holistic integrative approach. I was at Scripps integrated medicine in San Diego in La Jolla with Dr. Mimi Guarneri for maybe two years, and now I'm the Director of Integrated Medicine at NYU and very interested in whatever we can do to try to help people to understand that there's so much that they can do for themselves, both with lifestyle changes and also taking appropriate supplements and understanding.

I'll just make these four points, because I know you're totally on board with it. Every single patient, in fact a patient I just saw, I spend time talking about wellness, and I say that wellness is not the absence of disease. Being well for me there are four pillars. There are four important points. I always call them the four legs of a stool, and they all need to be intact and working properly for you to be well. One is nutrition with appropriate supplements. Two is exercise and flexibility. Three is stress management, and four is sleep. That's a quick summary of where I'm at.

Dr. Gould: That's a lot to say, and I'm glad that you did mention that. The whole aspect of wellness is something that I've been focusing on. A lot of people are starting to understand that in dentistry, as in any other profession, when it comes to someone's health being proactive and getting ahead of a problem before it starts is really critical, and I don't think I've heard anybody really explain wellness in such a concise way. Thank you for doing that. I appreciate it.

Which is going to bring us to your book *Magnificent Magnesium*. This isn't your new book, but this is how I found you. If found you through my work in sleep disordered breathing, and myself personally as a sleep apnea sufferer I came across the idea that magnesium would be a help for insomnia, and as I listened to some of your speaking engagements and read more I realized this is so much more than just another supplement that someone should be taking. What opened your eyes to magnesium? Was there an ah-ha moment where you said, I've got to focus on this?

Dr. Goodman: Good question, Joel. The question is why pick magnesium? I started to just hear about magnesium, because unfortunately we really don't talk about the stuff in medical school, even though mine goes way back. Even today nutrition is not a big subject. Even I'm talking to my colleagues about magnesium they kind of sometimes just don't get it. It's partly because you need a moment where you realize that this is such a crucial nutrient, and I always tell people seriously, if there's only one nutrient that you can take it should be magnesium.

I know Vitamin D is right up there, but I'm just saying because magnesium is not made by the body. You require it. You're require it from basically dietary intake. So there are over 300, probably 350, enzyme systems in the body that require magnesium. Essentially your body can't function properly if you're magnesium deficient. Where do you get magnesium? You get it from dark green leafy vegetables, nuts and seeds, halibut, Greek yogurt, some dairy products. The bottom line is people don't get enough of these vegetables, spinach, Swiss chard, broccoli, that type of stuff. Unfortunately even if they are eating that they may get the stuff from soil that is deficient in magnesium.

I actually learned measuring what I call red blood cell magnesium level on every single patient, because we don't have a good way to tell if you're magnesium deficient. Serum magnesium is not a good way. Only 1% of the magnesium in the body is in the serum, so when your doctor measures a serum magnesium he says you're okay, it doesn't mean you're okay, because the body does everything it can to keep that serum level in the normal range, even at the expense of tissue deficiency. I measure red blood cell magnesium. The best lab for it is Lab Corp, so you can ask your doctor for that. It's not perfect, but it's better, much better than the serum magnesium. I find that 75-80% of my patients are deficient, and they've got suboptimal levels. That goes along with other literature that says 80% of Americans are deficient in magnesium.

I know you know this, because you read my book, but there are major problems that occur when you're magnesium deficient. Let's start with the symptoms. How would people know just what symptoms may indicate? It doesn't mean you are, but may indicate. You can imagine it's a broad spectrum, because every system is affected. So the commonest symptoms I'm going to mention are fatigue, palpitations, muscle cramps, insomnia, anxiety, depression's associated with magnesium deficiency. Magnesium deficiency's associated with asthma, with diabetes, with obesity. Those last few are obviously conditions, but in terms of symptoms a lot of nonspecific symptoms, but I really cannot tell you how many times I've had patients come and go, "I'm sleeping well. My palpitations are gone. I don't have muscle cramps anymore. I feel much better. I feel much more energy." So those are symptoms.

Then if you wind up being chronically magnesium deficient you're at risk from these things that I spoke to you about, atherosclerosis and diabetes and obesity. The bottom line, Joel, is that most people are deficient. Because it's so easy to take magnesium, and it's so inexpensive I'm just going to make this last point, which is that everybody can take it except people who have kidney problems. So you do have to check with your doctor.

Dr. Gould: Before you get too far, the tests that you're talking about, and when it comes to testing for different things it's always confusing for most patients, even confusing for myself and other doctors. You're testing the actual content of magnesium in a red blood cell rather than in the tissue. Is that very usual?

Dr. Goodman: You separate the serum, right, from the red blood cells, so you actually have to spin it down to do it properly. What we're doing is we're getting content of magnesium that's not in the serum. The red cell is a very, as you can imagine, it's a metabolic powerhouse, the red blood cell. It's actually the supplier of oxygen to the tissues, hemoglobin. So we're getting a good sense with what's going on by just knowing how much magnesium there is in the red cells.

Dr. Gould: Right. Before you came on I made everybody go back to their high school days of ATP and the Krebs Cycle and things they didn't want to remember. So we did talk about that. The question I have is if someone is deficient how long does it take for them to build this? Is this something that builds within days or weeks or does it take two or three months like Vitamin D takes a while to build into your tissues?

Dr. Goodman: Good question. Just to go back to a point you made. ADP gets converted to ATP for energy to be utilized, and magnesium is a key cofactor for that. So it's very important that you have magnesium around so that you can convert ADP to ATP, which I'm sure is what you mentioned.

Here's the deal in terms of how long does it take. What I do know is that symptoms can improve very quickly. I've seen people come back a week later saying they feel a difference. I've seen a blood pressure drop significantly within two weeks. I don't measure red cell magnesium levels again before at least three months, because there's no point. I think that it takes a few weeks before you can expect to see an improvement in the red blood cell levels, but I don't pay huge attention to it, because sometimes the level doesn't increase significantly, yet the patient is feeling much better.

I use the red blood cell magnesium to help me diagnose a deficiency, and then I repeat it, but if I've got someone on a good amount of magnesium and they're feeling better, if the level is still on the low side I'm not going to start pushing up to really high doses. I don't believe it's a test that you've got to keep checking, but I do check it, and I have seen it improve significantly in people who are deficient.

Dr. Gould: I wanted to ask you. There's a way you can ingest magnesium, but there's also you can soak your feet in Epsom salts. There's an oil that you talk about that you can rub onto your body. Do you ingest any of that? Does that get into your red blood cells?

Dr. Goodman: Sure. That's a good question. You can get your magnesium through, obviously we spoke about the diet. Then you can get it through supplements that you're taking. Let's make a point about that. I always recommend taking a supplement of magnesium that ends in ate. For example, citrate, glycinate, threonate, malate, those are the best forms because they are the most bioavailable. Magnesium hydroxide is actually milk of magnesium, so if you go to the store, and you get a magnesium you'll end up probably getting magnesium hydroxide because it's the cheapest, and it doesn't have very good absorption. I always tell patients, unless you've got a problem with constipation, avoid the hydroxide form. I happen to like something called magnesium dimalate. It's a company called Jigsaw. The only reason I mention it is they have a slow release technology, and that means it's going to be slowly absorbed over several hours. That's better than getting a bolus into your stomach, and then you end up having an increased risk for GI side effects. That's the tablet form.

Then you can take it in the skin. You can actually use a spray, or you can actually use a lotion. There's a company called Ancient Minerals. I have nothing to do with these companies in terms of getting, I want you to know that. I mention them. I do not, and I'm saying this on the air, I'm not making any money because someone goes and buys these products. I happen just to think that they are available and that they're the best ones out there. Ancient Minerals is where you can get your lotions and sprays. Then I use Epsom salts. I have a bath approximately once a week, and it feels great, because it's another wonderful way. You put a cup of Epsom salts in a bath, and you soak for 15 minutes. You can just put your feet in if you don't like getting into a bath. Put your feet in a bowl with some Epsom salts. That's the transdermal way to do it.

Whichever way you're getting, it's just like rubbing in hormones. You can raise the levels of the red blood cells, whether it's coming in the red cells through the skin or whether you're getting it through the gut.

Dr. Gould: I want to interrupt you for one second just to let my listeners know, because we are live that we're going to go a
bit over in time, just because we got a bit delayed. If you
still have a few minutes there's a few more things I want
to talk about. I wanted to let everybody listening know
that we're just going to go a bit over. I want to go back to
this. First of all, when we're done here we're going to tell
everybody about your website and how they can order
your book and how they can get more information on
this. I will be providing information that we talked today on my website, so people who want to know where
they can get these different compounds can look to
that. So we'll talk about that later. Just anybody listening who's interested, we will have that for a follow up.

The one issue that we sort of haven't covered is the
stomach or the GI upset that people who just start
taking magnesium have. Is that avoided by doing the
transdermal method?

Dr. Goodman: Yes. That's absolutely right, Joel. You're not going to have
that side effect if you take it transdermally. I haven't experienced any problems. That's why I tell people with
any magnesium that you take by mouth you may get
some loose stool effect. So whatever amount you're taking try to cut it back. For example, I think we should
mention what's a good dose. People don't know. I tell
them a good starting dose is 3mg per pound. Most of
my female patients are on 400mg a day. My male patients 500mg a day. You can actually take up to easily
5mg per pound. If you're stressed you should increase
your level to 5mg per pound.

You can take it if you have insomnia problems all at
night. I've had a lot of patients who just by taking the
whole dose, let's say the 500mg at night before they go
to sleep, because it helps you to sleep. You can do that,

or you can divide it in two or three doses. If there's a loose stool effect, you can cut it down to even once a day. Obviously it's better than nothing, but then I tell people you may not be getting enough. You would have to supplement transdermally, and I want to go back to this idea of having this magnesium dimalate slow release is a good way to really minimize the chances of loose stools and diarrhea.

Dr. Gould: That's actually what I was pretty interested in. Just because we've got a lot of people with gastrointestinal issues in general. I want to switch gears real quick here. I'm just kind of curious. To me, when I read your work it was a profound understanding, because I'm all about intervening with getting a good cleaning before you get periodontal disease, but to me this seemed like such a no-brainer. It seemed like such a basic thing that an element that's such a huge part of who we are as humans. What are your colleagues saying about this? Is this something that's being received well? How has it gone?

Dr. Goodman: That's a good question, and the answer is I wish it was better. I can tell you that I'm part of a preventative medicine team at NYU, and I can tell you the good news. The good news is they invited me to come and give a talk about magnesium, and I spoke to them with a fellow. We prepared it, and they are at least saying, let's hear about it. Some of them have actually emailed me and said to me, how much should we take and what should we tell the patient? So it's kind of hush hush, because it's not easy for people to accept this and take it on board easily when it hasn't been drummed into us. Why is that? There's so much literature. You saw in my book how many articles I quoted, but a lot of them are observational studies, and there's so much information. Until a lot of traditional physicians see some double blind randomized trial in a big journal they don't believe that this is for real, and I tell people, please have an open mind. At least try it on the patients. You'll be amazed just how much improvement you actually see.

I work with a chief of psychiatry. He's in my office here at NYU. He does a session here, and he told me next year he's doing a whole session, a whole morning, on holistic integrative approaches to psychiatric illness, and he asked me to speak about magnesium. So your question is a very good one. I think that we are making progress. You've got to start with people who've got an open mind who want to listen, and slowly but surely we educate each other. I've tried to think of myself as a bridge, Joel, just like you, between traditional and alternative and integrative medicine. We've got to have a communication going on before we can even begin to hope the other side's going to take anything on board, and we have problem like, as you know, on the other side where you've got some people saying that everything the doctors do with pharmaceuticals is giving poison, which is ridiculous. We've got the extremists on both sides.

Dr. Gould: It brings me back to we had a conversation that neither one of us have come up initial in the American system, and we maybe have a different perspective. One of the things that as a Canadian working here I get frustrated because on one hand we have the absolute must have a double blind study done by a reputable university before they'll even look at something that's natural, and on the other hand we have the farthest everything raw, just the whole everything is holistic, everything is not based in science. I don't like that fringe either. I know there's a middle ground, and I'm here with this show hopefully raising awareness about someone like you and your book, because this is obvious to me that there's a very easy middle ground. It's having a background in science and being open to the idea that we are animals that evolved over the last million years, and we have to look at our environment and what we ate to make us whole.

I'm glad to have somebody like you on my show. I want to wind things up here. I do want to have the opportunity, because I do want to talk to you for future about K2, and I'd love to talk to you about some other things.

Dr. Goodman: Sure.

Dr. Gould: For today, I want to let all my listeners know, if you would give us your website, and again, his books are available on Amazon.com, of course. We will have the links on my website. I'll go ahead and let you tell everybody how to get a hold of you, and we'll let you go. I know you've probably had a long day, and you're probably ready to relax.

Dr. Goodman: I'm not quite done yet. It's like the middle of my day. My website's DennisGoodmanMD.com, and you'll find an email address there. I'm at NYU. You can find me if you just go and Google my name, Dennis Goodman, MD, you'll find all the information. I've written three books. One's magnesium, one Vitamin K2, another one was about krill and omega 3s. I'm working on my next book, and my whole idea that we're educated, and I commend you too, Joel, because we're trying to raise awareness. We're trying to give people information, and some of the information we have maybe it's not steeped in the science that other people expect. It doesn't mean you don't want to listen and say let's see how it works, as long as it's not doing any harm. I am pushing all the time to do studies, to try to have a scientific approach, because we want to be able to make recommendations that are not just empiric stories. I know you believe the same thing. My website is DennisGoodmanMD.com. My email is Dennis.Goodman@NYUMC.org, but you can find that information on my website.

Dr. Gould: Thank you so much. You're such an articulate guest. I can't wait to have you back in the future.

Dr. Goodman: I look forward to it, and congratulations on what you do, because until people can get out there and speak out it people don't know. We didn't get to this, but one of the reasons we don't have these big studies is because it's very expensive, right? Unfortunately only the drug companies can afford these very expensive studies. So we've got to try very hard to find ways that we can do proper studies without spending too much money.

Dr. Gould: I totally agree. Thank you so much. You have a great rest of your day.

Dr. Goodman: Take care. Bye bye.

Dr. Gould: Bye. All right, everybody, that was Dr. Dennis Goodman. Really groundbreaking stuff here. Thank you for listening. We ran a bit late, but I think it was well worth it. Please with any type of vitamin supplements for any medical issue please consult with your own doctors. This show is for informational purposes only. Let's be reasonable. You can always contact me through my Facebook page or on Twitter and at ModernAmericanDentistry.com, and I'll be happy to answer any of your questions. Thank you so much, and until next week, get your smile on. Stay well. Thank you.

GYSO – Eps. 9
Dr. Satsha Gominak Vitamin D
and Sleep Apnea

Dr. Gould: Welcome to Get Your Smile On. This is your wellness dentist, Dr. Joel Gould, here with another episode of Get Your Smile On. We are broadcasting live from beautiful Manhattan Beach, California. Tonight we are on early. We usually go on at 7:00PM. We are on at 5:00PM for several different reasons, most importantly, my guest tonight is Dr. Satsha Gominak. Dr. Gominak, are you out there?

Dr. Gominak: Thank you for inviting me.

Dr. Gould: My pleasure. Sorry for the technical difficulties. Broadcasting and computers, there are some issues when you go live, but I think we're all good. Usually I start off this show and talk about what the topic is, and you and I talked about what I wanted to call this episode, and I thought the idea of calling it Escape Permanent Winter would be a pretty good one. Before we get into that I would love you to introduce yourself and tell us a little bit about yourself, your education, and where you're at now.

Dr. Gominak: Joel, thank you very much for inviting me to take part in your podcast. I am a neurologist. I practice in Tyler, Texas. I'm originally from California. I went to college at UC Santa Barbara, and then I did medical school in Texas. So I'm actually very happy in both California and Texas, and currently I'm mostly interested in improving my patients' sleep. I've practiced for 30 years, and I have a general neurology practice, because of a couple of unusual accidental discoveries I'm now able to improve my patients' sleep, and that's what interests me the most. That's why we're having this discussion today.

Dr. Gould: Fantastic. Initially I became aware of you when I found out, for myself having a wellness dentistry podcast I sort of on my first podcast defined what that means, but anything related to health. After 25 years in dentistry I was having some personal physical problems that had to do with my sleep. I have sleep apnea, and I found out also that I'm terribly Vitamin D deficient. Initially you came to me by way of my sleep apnea research, and I saw one of your first lectures on YouTube 2013 where you started to talk about Vitamin D and a whole bunch of different things. I guess we want to just cut right to the chase here, and let's talk about Vitamin D. We talked in past shows that Vitamin D is not a Vitamin, it's actually a hormone. What I want to talk to you about, if you want to maybe sort of briefly describe how you came upon the whole D issue?

Dr. Gominak: I would say that most of the things we're going to talk about tonight are accidental occurrences in my practice that then I try to figure out an explanation for. What happened to me was I had five years of doing sleep studies in young, healthy women who came to see me for headaches, and most of them did not have sleep apnea. Most of them just did not have enough rapid eye movement sleep, and many of them just couldn't sleep. Many of them were so sleep deprived that there was no point in even doing a sleep study. They could tell me they didn't sleep at all. So I had a population that was very different than the group of patients who had been originally described, which were overweight males after heart surgery who stopped breathing in the ICU when they were sitting bolt upright.

Because I had a group of patients who had much milder disease, they provided me with a lot of challenges. For instance, if you don't have sleep apnea, what do you do to help them? If they sleep for many hours but don't get into deeper phases of sleep, what should I do to help them? Ultimately, there are no medicines that actually replicate normal sleep. There are things that coax us into sleep and to some extent copy the light sleep, but nothing that really gets us into deep sleep. So I was left with a lot of frustration, a lot of patients who I felt I could probably make them better if I could make their sleep better.

Mostly my question was why is it that everyone I do a sleep study on, and now I've stopped doing them just on my headache patients and I'm doing them on anybody who comes in who'll let me do a sleep study, and I wind up doing sleep studies on 8 year olds and 88 year olds, and they're all abnormal. To me that was shocking, Number 1, and Number 2, very upsetting because I had very little to offer. I had sleeping pills, and I had C-PAP masks, pressure masks that you strap on your face, which are obviously not normal. It's what we had, but it really won't help someone who doesn't stop breathing. All that mask does is push air in to try to keep the airway open.

About five years into doing all these sleep studies I had a young 18 year old who had a sleep study that showed she was in light sleep, which means she was sleeping, but she wasn't getting into the phases where she made repairs to her body. She was sleeping for 10 hours, but no deep sleep was recorded, and that was shocking, and she was otherwise a normal 18 year old. She wound up having a B12 deficiency. The only reason why I tested that was because she asked me what she should do now that she was so tired, and I really just said, who does tired labs? I really had no idea what they were, and she turned out to have a B12 that was very low.

Because her sleep study was so abnormal, and because

the B12 was so low, for the first time I began to think about wouldn't this be an exciting idea that we could give back a vitamin which would be a raw material that these cells in the brain stem need in order to make the transitions into deeper sleep. So this would be something we could give the patient back again, and they might sleep normally. It was just a totally foreign idea, and I began to measure B12 levels on my patients.

Soon after that one of my patients mentioned Vitamin D and that her doctor had measured her Vitamin D, gave her Vitamin D, her wrist pain got better. Because I was already drawing blood I threw in the Vitamin D level, not really being that interested in it, thinking it had to do with bone pain, because I was as misinformed as everyone else. Then over a period of about four months I began to realize that every single person I did a Vitamin D level on it was low.

Then by complete accident I happened to give a low dose, but in two patients who were wearing C-PAP masks successfully, who had pretty high D levels, and they got better. They came back and said, this C-PAP mask didn't really do anything for me. It did not take my headaches away, but that little message that you sent me about the Vitamin D made my sleep better within about three weeks. Two people came back in a week and told me that. Then after that very few other few other people got better.

There was a long process of trying to figure out why these two guys got better. Why is it that the dosing is so wrong? Then after that there's a huge body of literature that shows that Vitamin D affects the parts of the brain stem that fascinate me about the control of keeping the airway open and keeping the timing of sleep correct. So there was a linkage in the literature, scientific literature, that was well documented that apparently had been completely ignored. It was already there, but no one had written about sleep and why it would be within this bigger picture of what Vitamin D does for us as an endocrine hormone.

Dr. Gould: I want to interrupt you there for a couple reasons. First of all, that's an incredible linking of sleep and Vitamin D, but I want to just sort of let my listeners understand what's so important about sleep. I know this is tough, because this is a shorter interview here, but I would love you to tell from a neurologist's point of view what sleep is. What's so important about it? I know this is a tough one, because I'll get you to sort of explain how this sort of comes out in the long run, but if you want to just generally talk about sleep, and then towards the end of what sleep does then we can talk about the release of hormones, because I think that where I'm seeing a lot of my patients who actually have sleep disorders is that the biggest issue is they're not necessarily understanding that the control of their entire bodies and the repair is so related to sleep. I guess we'll call it the elevator pitch on why sleep is so important and what happens when we don't have it.

Dr. Gominak: Okay. That's a very good question, Joel. I have to tell you that the first part of this is to understand that humans are here, animals are here, living things are here, on the planet with no users' manual. That's a very different concept than the way I present myself as a physician. I walk in the room. I have a white coat on. I try to present myself as being all-knowing, but in actual fact medicine is an observation, and therefore it's always changing. Our interpretation of it is always changing. What I'm going to tell you about my interpretation of what we do in sleep is based on for 10 years listening to people who don't sleep normally, and then putting it together.

In my view, the body is being used up for 18 hours, and then we lay down, and we repair. We make every chemical we need. We make little packets of each chemical, insulin, serotonin, dopamine, our own Xanax like chemicals. We make little packets with those chemicals, and we store them in the cell so that after 8 hours of sleeping we can wake up, and we have all the chemicals we need to be awake for another 16 or 18 hours. That is not the way we are told about sleep, because currently the best anybody says about sleep is we really don't know what it's for. From my point of view, I know what it's for. We either use the body up, or we repair it. If we don't repair it, and we don't make the chemicals we need, we all feel terrible. My practice is filled with people who have not slept normally for 2, 5, 10, 30 years. Then I watch what happens to them if they don't go into the reparative phases of sleep.

In retrospect, my view of it is all the repair mechanisms that we describe in medicine, whether it's how does the pancreas make enough insulin to last the whole day? How does my GI tract work? How does it repair itself? How do nerves repair themselves? Everything that I've read about how we repair the body probably only happens while we're sleeping. There's a very important reason for that. When you open up certain proteins in each cell that enable a cell to repair itself, so it has to make repair chemicals, and it has to make proteins, and it has to build things within that cell. In order to build itself again, you actually have to open up processes that would allow the cell to actually, if it were not tightly supervised, if the brain weren't paying complete attention to that process, if you let it go a little unsupervised that cell could decide it not only wanted to repair itself, but it wanted to grow an entire human being.

That means these repair processes open up the potential for growth and then cancer and things that would go haywire, every single night. So I think the entire brain is extremely involved in supervising every single piece of the body's repair. Every part of the brain has an assigned toenail, knee, internal organ, that it is responsible for supervising the repair processes while we are sleeping. If you do not have that every night, the body begins to age faster than the people around you. This is now an epidemic, and most of our population is aging faster.

Dr. Gould: That brings up a couple of great points. First of all I just want to point out that when we talk about cancer what we're talking about is a bunch of cells that aren't supposed to be growing in the right location that start to grow. That's a basic description of it. The sleep actually helps our immune system to also protect us from those type of issues by taking care of our white blood cells. The connection with the Vitamin D as well as the repair mechanism for our chromosomes, do you think that's highly related to sleep, or is that a coincidence?

Dr. Gominak: They're absolutely related. The hardest part about Vitamin D is that it is active on multiple levels. So if you open a textbook, or if you look in the internet, and you ask, "What is the mechanism of Vitamin D?" you will actually see that Vitamin D and A and several other things are pivotal to going into the nucleus of the cell, the actual DNA protective mechanism that keeps the DNA coiled and quiet until we need it is opened. The A and D and several other cofactors sit on the actual chromosomes and help to express certain proteins. That's one mechanism.

It turns out that Vitamin D has multiple layers of mechanisms. It's a single chemical that actual does something different for a red blood cell than it does a brain cell, and there are Vitamin D receptors in certain cells in the brain stem where the Vitamin D probably has a slightly different affect than this expression of proteins. That means that Vitamin D is affecting the body in multiple different ways, which is one of the reasons why it's such a confusing literature.

The thing that I feel is different about my viewpoint is I went into this literature asking, is this possibly why the entire planet stopped sleeping normally when electricity arrived 50 years ago? The question that I posed was different.

Dr. Gould: This is probably a perfect opportunity just to get back to the D. We'll finish up with the sleep. Without proper sleep our bodies basically go into dysfunction, and it can affect anyone differently. Part of what you're saying also is that for people who are getting terrible sleep that if they have genetic predisposition to a certain type of disease that, because their bodies aren't healthy, that disease is going to get expressed. An easy example is that I have Crohn's disease. We talked that I probably had a Vitamin D deficiency my entire life, since I grew up in Canada, and it's pretty dark up there, and I didn't eat much, other than probably candies and cookies. So my ability to fight it off, or my ability for my intestines and my whole system to work probably were interrupted by having a low Vitamin D, and in my case also sleep issues as well that were probably related.

Dr. Gominak: Yes. They are related. I like what you said. One of the difficult parts is that when you take someone's sleep away they only manifest the diseases they have a genetic predilection for. That means you can't think of it as we're going to make you not sleep, and then everybody will get the same thing. They don't. they'll get things that run in their family. That's kind of complicated.

Dr. Gould: I think that this is both the most complex thing in the world and also the most simple. The whole story is that we talked about, so if we're chronically Vitamin D deficient as a population, and we talked in a previous podcast episode about how the farther you get away from the 30th parallel the more disease that you have, and it's probably related to Vitamin D. What you have done is you've recommended supplementing people's Vitamin D until they get up to what we would consider an evolutionary level, as if we actually lived outside. Let's just talk about the Vitamin D, because it's a hormone it has to be calibrated or titrated, as we say in the medical field. You had recommended to your patients a zone to be in. What is that zone?

Dr. Gominak: The zone is 60-80, and that's a blood measurement. That grows out of asking more than 2,000 people how do you feel? How's your sleep? There has been no single article before our published article that asked that question. It has been very consistent now over five years that when you ask a patient how they feel, and once their Vitamin D crosses 60 their sleep is different. Almost everyone at the beginning can tell a difference in how they feel. So between 60 and 80 the patient's sleep is good. Within the first year probably at least three quarters of the patients will be able to recognize when their sleep changes if their Vitamin D goes too high or too low.

Dr. Gould: I just want to break in there. For the average person, I went to my doctor, and I said, "I'm turning a certain age, and I want to get whatever tests I need to get done." I specifically asked about my Vitamin D. What was interesting is that he said, "Your Vitamin D is normal. You're great." I asked him, "What is normal?" He said, "You're 20." I had already been taking Vitamin D supplements at that point in time. So that was me with taking some supplements. We're talking that the ideal would probably be somewhere between 60 to 80.

Dr. Gominak: Yes. You were really badly off.

Dr. Gould: Yes. Not only that, but the most important part of that is that my doctor, he's a good guy, but he's basing what he's telling me on what he sees out there in the literature. He says, "No, your D is fine." He thinks that that's okay. The take home message for me is that not only do we have a problem that we're deficient of Vitamin D, but we have a medical industry that doesn't necessarily know what to tell you. When I ask my patients, and I say, "Tell me about your Vitamin D," and they say, "I'm fine. I take supplements." I say, "What are you taking?" "I take 1,000 international units." Everyone has a very unusual idea of what good D is and what their D's supposed to be, but this is seemingly one of the most critical things in the current modern health.

Dr. Gominak: I agree with you.

Dr. Gould: We're going to go on just a bit here. We talked about the whole idea that these are modern sicknesses. These are the restless leg syndrome, the fibromyalgia, migraines, stuff that you're seeing on a regular basis. We didn't see this 40 years ago or 50 years ago, did we?

Dr. Gominak: I don't think that they were epidemic 30 or 40 or 50 years ago. The way I present this to my patients, because I got so paranoid at the beginning of this, because every week I would come up with something else that was linked to Vitamin D deficiency, and not only would my patients think that's weird, I think it's weird. So I kept thinking there's no way that all of these things can be linked to Vitamin D deficiency, but they are. What I came up with as an explanation was I don't have a drug to give you to keep that hand from growing out of your chest. I don't see any patients come into the office with a hand growing out of their chest. I don't have any patients like that. Therefore, the only thing that medicine really reacts to and makes up stories about is what walks in the door.

The other thing my office isn't filled with are patients with syphilis, patients with diphtheria, patients with tuberculosis, patients with polio, patients that would have filled my office in 1910 we have actually cured those illnesses. So what I actually am observing is this patient population. I'm sitting there. They make appointments. They walk in, and I ask them what's bothering them, and there's a whole list and then over the last 50 years we think that that list is "normal" because it's so common.

I realized in about the third month of reading about the Vitamin D that I actually thought it was normal and laudable medicine the internist sending me a patient who's 40 years old who's on four pills. I thought that was good medicine. There's a little something for antidepressant, something for reflux. They're on a little because their feet hurt, or their back hurts. They're on something else for their allergies. I realized that as a 40 year old myself when I was 40, I didn't take any pills. Not only that, I as a 60 year old really don't want to take any pills. I really don't want to go see the doctor. That means there really is a weird assumption that I think it's normal that a human being at 40 years old should have daily headache, back pain, allergies, problems with their bowels, and reflux, and be pretty depressed and anxious. Yet I think that's normal because it is so common.

Now I think of it in a different way, and I think these are all the things that have resulted in the population because we missed something. We really did cure polio and diphtheria and syphilis, but we missed this one thing that is pivotal, and therefore the population that is around me, including me, is suffering from things that are all connected like spokes on a wheel to this one major hormone that we missed that turns out to run sleep. We have also left sleep for last, because doctors are human. We are unconscious during the time we're sleeping. We haven't really had a window into it. So the D and the sleep have been left for last.

Dr. Gould: This is like the last frontier. What's really funny is that when I was sleeping I would wake up every morning feeling a certain way, and what I realized after getting my D up higher is that when you're used to crummy sleep, when you're used to the way you feel, it seems normal. This is normal to a lot of people how they feel.

This is a perfect opportunity to discuss, the way I describe this is we took an incredibly highly evolved mammal, the human, and we put it into a beautiful air-conditioned, gilded cage. It's getting in the sick in the same way that when we take a whale and put it into captivity it's going to get sick too, because it doesn't have the actual conditions that it grew up on evolutionarily speaking. All these modern diseases, these are a result of taking this human animal out of its environment and putting it into a way more comfortable one.

I don't want to go back to living in a cave, but I feel completely different even three, four weeks into having myself treated for sleep apnea. I'm now getting a full night's sleep, and I'm getting my Vitamin D up. Just my feeling alone is pretty incredible. The issue that has come up is this sounds so wacky that it could just be something as simple as this, but it's kind of true. What do your colleagues think about this idea that maybe we don't have to give a pill for every single thing according to what the pharmaceutical companies want us to do? What do your colleagues think about what you're doing?

Dr. Gominak: I think the way you presented that you became interested in this because you weren't feeling well, that is the pivotal place. Number 1, I've hit a wall with my colleagues, and now I don't even try to talk to them about it, but when someone doesn't feel well, especially when they don't sleep, so when a physician doesn't sleep well, and they stumble on my literature, or they're sending me patients and I send them information back, what I'm doing with their patient is something that they wonder about about their own health, they become very interested in it. It really has to be through their own physical experience of not sleeping well, and those people are then invested in kind of breaking out of this idea that all of medicine has already been discovered.

All of us who go to medical school think that everything we learned there was the truth. Oddly, for the physicians, I'm 60, my physicians in my age group thought that fibromyalgia, chronic fatigue, and sleep apnea were really made up diagnoses. A lot of us thought they were just totally created out of nothing, because they weren't in our medical school classes. Because there hasn't really been a good firm pathophysiology, or how does sleep apnea really arise? How does fibromyalgia arise? Nobody really knows that. I think I do, but what's written about it is so unsatisfying to the patient and to the physicians that we still kind of left those as, I kind of believe in them and I kind of don't.

As soon as you have nonrestorative sleep yourself, there is a huge drive to try to figure that out. You realize that your illness is related to that, and all of a sudden it becomes the most important thing you could possibly learn about. My colleagues that are suffering from it are very motivated, and they will sit and listen. The ones that have missed that idea, or just last night I was asking another physician, a guy who's wearing a C-PAP mask and has never thought further past that, hasn't thought about the fact that my cat doesn't wear a C-PAP mask, neither do the squirrels. Nobody else is wearing a C-PAP mask except human beings. Only doctors would come up with something that crazy.

You know what's interesting about that? I don't actually make fun of a patient who has to have their C-PAP mask on. They've become addicted to it, yet I'm not derisive of them. That's a very interesting thing, because I'm derisive, all of medicine is derisive of the people who need sleeping pills, as though there's something badly wrong with them. There's something inherently weak about them. We don't treat people who use C-PAP masks in the same way, yet we should.

Dr. Gould: Interesting. The thing I'm seeing here, I'm seeing two types of patients in my practice, which is interesting. I'm seeing the female patient who's done everything and feels terrible, and when I come in and look in their mouth and I see all this obvious signs to me of sleep apnea, because the signs in the mouth they jump out at you if someone's been sick for a while. They are so grateful and so interested they can't wait to do a sleep study, and they can't believe that no one's ever suggested this before, because their sleep is terrible, and they admit it.

The second thing that kind of scares me is I've got plenty of patients who are already on a C-PAP, and the way the medical system works is that once you get a C-PAP you're out the door, and nobody's checking on you. I'm screening these patients with their C-PAP machines, and I can tell you that a lot of them are not functional. They're not calibrated correctly. I'm seeing all kinds of stuff that kind of scares me.

So the whole idea that you get diagnosed with sleep apnea, you get a C-PAP machine, you're stuck with it your entire life, and no one ever checks you again I think is crazy and ridiculous. There is so many things that I've just discovered in the last little while that are actually crazy and ridiculous. This whole situation with sleep apnea and, again, Vitamin D.

I want to turn things just real quick. We talked about this is tough one, because it's really complex. What struck me when I heard you first speak is you said, "Vitamins, I don't care about vitamins." I thought the same thing. I'm interested in real stuff, and I think that vitamins are flaky and silly, but what I want to share with my listeners is the whole permanent winter idea that if our bodies are deficient of sleep and Vitamin D our bodies think that we're in a whole different time zone. We're hibernating. I guess, maybe this is going to be tough for you to explain, but if you could explain the whole Vitamin D and why you need B vitamins as well.

First of all, I just want to take this opportunity to say that this show is for informational purposes. Do not go out and do anything crazy. Please consult with your physician or your dentist or me, even email me, before you do anything crazy. However, you can out into the sun and get Vitamin D safely if you know how to do it. I'm not worried about that. Tell us about the difference between somebody who's D deprived versus somebody who's got full D, and what's the difference between their digestive system and how they are as a human?

Dr. Gominak: The first interesting part is that the linkage of Vitamin D to multiple systems in the body, and how it fits together to explain how every animal on the planet can put up with a winter and a summer was all summarized by a gentleman named Walter Stump, who was a steroid chemist. He started publishing in the late 80s, and he has 20 years of articles that describe why we would have a hormone that we make on our skin that in humans is absorbed through the skin, but in all other furry animals, so pigs and humans absorb it through the skin, probably reptiles do too, but mammals that are furry actually lick the Vitamin D that's made in their fur, so it actually goes in orally, which is one of the confusing aspects. This is a hormone. We make it on our skin. We actually make it, but it can come in orally.

The first original mistake was made because we do most of our experimentation on rats, because rats are nocturnal that means they have actually adapted a Vitamin D receptor that can take a similar hormone, it's not the same, but it's similar. It's called D2, unfortunately it's still being given as a prescription, but D2 is made by a fungus that grows on grain. That means that we use these animals that could be kept in a cage inside as our model, missing the fact that 10 years later there was a similar but not identical chemical described on the skin of pigs that had been left in the sun. Dr. Stump took all of this information, put it together, and made a beautiful explanation for the reason why we have a hormone that is linked to our level of metabolism, i.e. it changes our thyroid hormone, it changes how much we eat, it is linked to whether or not we are in the mode to put on weight, just like bears.

As bears reach the end of the season they put on weight so that they can hibernate in the winter. They use the fat stores to get through the winter. That is run not voluntarily by the bear. The bear doesn't just decide its going to lay in the ground. There are hormonal frameworks that cause that bear to actually go into a sleep mode that lasts for months on end. Humans do the same thing, run by the same set of hormones. We actually get up every 24 hours, but in the past in order to survive long winters, periods of time when there would be no food for weeks on end were survivable because we would sleep for long periods, because we would actually use our fat stores in much the same way as a bear did.

Because we are no longer thinking of ourselves in that way, medicine has missed the fact that there is a hormone that connects all of that. One of the fascinating things for me is the gastroenterology literature that has moved in the last 30 years that I've been interested in neurology, they've been studying what happens in the GI tract, and during the last 10 years where I've been studying sleep they've been studying who are the bacteria that live in our colon. There's a whole body of literature that talks about the fact that the wrong intestinal bacteria are epidemic throughout all the developed countries, in the same patient populations that have sleep apnea. There's a link in terms of the appearance of when this epidemic occurred, and within the same populations, and there is multiple parts of the literature that substantiate the idea that many of the autoimmune diseases are patients who have the wrong bacteria in their colon.

The cause and effect has not been clear. What happened to me was I'm interested in D. I'm not interested in poop, but it turns out one of the things that doesn't get better when the D is perfect is the patients don't lose weight. They're still fat. I know that they gain weight because they were D deficient, but when I get the D perfect for two years they still don't lose weight. Most of the patients who had irritable bowel at the end of two years they had perfect D levels, their sleep's better, they still have irritable bowel. That didn't get better. There were two or three things that were left over at the end of two years. The third one was terrible pain. Many of my patients had gotten better, yet they still had back pain, leg pain, knee pain, joint pain, muscle pain, a lot of pain that was unexplained.

By weird accident, one of my patients walked in with a book on a B vitamin. I still had no interest in vitamins. I still really was just interested in Vitamin D, but my patients were failing. There were still things that weren't fixed, and because she brought me this book I happened to say, this is interesting. It's a B vitamin that's linked to pain. It's a B vitamin that makes joint pain go away, and this B vitamin, called pantothenic acid, makes cortisol. That would link to all the joint pain that all my patients have that's unexplained. She says in this book that pantothenic acid is pivotal in sleep. It makes the patients sleep better.

I think, I like the idea, but why would the patients be B deficient? I'm still operating in the same mindset as everybody else. I eat well. I do what my doctor tells me. If you eat a good diet, you don't have to take B vitamins. I don't really like taking vitamins. I'm very self-conscious about giving them to my patients, because so many of my colleagues think I'm a wacko now. It leads down a road that happens to lead me to this B vitamin that turns out to be only probably made by our intestinal bacteria, which then becomes, this is weird here's a vitamin that's made by our intestinal bacteria, and all of us have the wrong ones, and we probably don't have any of that vitamin anymore.

So it leads me into a second set of vitamins, and another discovery, which is if the B vitamins are all made daily, or have to be eaten daily, and are peed out on that day and can't be stored, how does that bear lie in the ground for six months and not eat and not die? Because the bacteria that eat his colonic mucus that that bear makes as their food supply lives inside him as the normal bacterial culture, which has always sustained that species for billions of years over multiple months. Those bacteria make the B vitamins. What that means is humans were never made to take vitamins. The animals were all here before the doctors came.

The odd part that is we all are in fact vitamin deficient now, and it was a cascade like a domino effect of the D, turns out our D feeds the intestinal bacteria. They need our D to have a certain makeup of species. Those species that are high D summer species make us put our calories into muscle, so we can plant 40 acres and actually be able to pick 40 acres of cotton in the summer. In the winter the population changes, because there's a low D, and low D favors other bacteria that make us take the few calories we eat and put it into fat. So you can watch all the epidemics forming in unison, the obesity, the sleep apnea, the colonic microbiome, and the chronic pain all growing starting in the late 70s and becoming now epidemic. It's not just the US. It's any country where air-conditioning has arrived. The countries where they do not have electricity do not have these epidemics in the same amount.

Dr. Gould: I'm going to stop you there. I want to recap what you're saying here, but we're going to take a very short break for one second, and we're going to come right back, and I want us to review that. I want to give that point back to my listeners and make sure that I understand exactly what you're saying. Hang on for one quick second, and we'll be right back.

Dr. Gominak: Okay.

Dr. Gould: Apparently we are not going to be taking a break. Are you still there?

Dr. Gominak: I'm still here.

Dr. Gould: Okay. We're going to continue on. I'm not really sure what happened there, but to recap, what you're saying is as the sun gets lower in the sky, as humans our intestinal bacteria started to change for winter, and instead of burning calories and building muscle we started putting on fat, to the point at which when I go to the gym, and I see all these people who are trying to lose some weight. They're struggling to the best of their abilities, but their body would actually prefer to burn their muscle than give up the fat, because their intestines say, winter's coming. Your intestine doesn't know that you're taking a flight to Hawaii, and you want to look good in your bikini. Your body just says, if I lose this fat I'm going to die, so I've got to do everything in my power not to burn my fat. I'm going to burn the muscle before I burn fat.

Dr. Gominak: That's correct.

Dr. Gould: So when I say we're all stuck in permanent winter, basically because of our intestinal bacteria, the ones that should be producing vitamins that give us growth and strength, we're hanging on to the ones that cause us to store fat and, no matter how hard we try. I guess, again, I see those people in the gym, and now knowing what I know I feel terrible. I want to say, slow down, because everything you're doing is right. Exercise is great, but you've got the wrong chemicals. You've got the wrong stuff going on.

Dr. Gominak: That's true. And they get hurt, and they feel worse. They can't lose weight, and they get so discouraged, and they come into see me, and I, as the physician, here's what I have to say to them. "Your back hurts because you're fat. Your feet hurt because you're fat. Everything hurts because of you. You're doing it wrong."

Dr. Gould:　　It's all your fault.

Dr. Gominak:　I think that is the wrong message, and I think that's a very discouraging message. I think that that's absolutely wrong. It's not their fault.

Dr. Gould:　　We get to this weird thing about sleep apnea, and it's like a shame thing. I just wrote an article about sleep apnea, and I had to admit, when I ask my patients, "Have you been tested for sleep apnea?" They just say, "I don't have it." It's a defensive mechanism, like I'm accusing them of being fat. It's really terrible.

I'm so glad that we sort of got to talk about this, because to me just the whole idea that we're all running around with the absolute wrong intestinal bacteria to make us the way we want to be, which is healthy, I don't think my intestines know that there's a 24 hour Ralph's around the corner from where I live, that I don't need to have extra fat stored on me, because I can just go down to In-N-Out Burger if I'm really desperate.

Dr. Gominak:　Yes. Let me add one other thing that's really interesting. There are now really good articles that describe that these bacteria, the winter bacterial population, actually make these short chain fatty acids, these little tiny chemicals, that then go into our bloodstream, and they go up in our nose, and they hit these little receptors that makes us want high calorie, high fat, high carbohydrate foods. It actually changes our appetite.

Dr. Gould:　　I guess the whole food industry is playing on that with our sweet and salty and all that stuff. It's pretty incredible stuff. Your concept of this, does anyone else understand it? Is this a school of thought anywhere that this is going on? To me, it's so simple that it makes absolute perfect sense. Is there a school of thought? Is there a group of doctors who are saying, this is the way it is, let's focus on this?

Dr. Gominak: No. That's the short answer. I and Walter Stump wrote the first and only article hypothesizing the idea that Vitamin D was linked to sleep apnea. There are multiple clinical trials ongoing, and there are clinical trials that substantiate that now that are prospective trials. I will be publishing soon the second part of this, which is it's not D. It is the effect on the intestinal bacteria, and that you can correct the intestinal bacteria and get your intestinal bacteria back into the summer mode, but in order to do that you have to give it lots of Vitamin D and lots of Bs, all of the Bs together. That's a difficult concept, and it's a new idea. What I've stepped into is there are about five new ideas that are linked together, and that means that it's very difficult for routine medical doctors to understand it. The ones that are suffering, the doctors that are sick, see that they have many of these things occurring in their body, but at the moment no one else, I do have other doctors like you who have looked at this and said, I want to do that, but you and I and Dr. Park are beginning that group of physicians.

Dr. Gould: I'm so glad to hear that. We're approaching the end of the show, and I want to review a few things for people, because there were so many really important points going on here. First of all, just before we leave that one point, this is definitely something that I'm so interested in, and the idea that we can do this, we can change our physiology by just doing very simple stuff just blows my mind. Anybody out there listening, you probably at some point soon can come to my website and get a little more understanding of how this is done with more detail. I try to keep this show sort of more simple, just not to get too confusing.

Real quick, I just want to review. Basically our major

issues are not getting enough sleep, because when we sleep that's when our bodies repair everything, and from that everything falls apart there. The Vitamin D is the critical piece of this, although it's much more complex. That'd be correct?

Dr. Gominak: That's correct, and let me just add that the last several years that I'm doing this I have become extremely respectful of these chemicals that I thought were trivial. I think, vitamins can kill you. Vitamins can give you terrible pain. Vitamins can be the actual reason why people wind up in the hospital with a stroke. No one sees it that way but me, but that's because I'm thinking of the effect of the vitamin on the sleep. Vitamins are only good for you if you need them. They are not good for you if you don't need them.

Ultimately, all of us would like to go back to the state where, just like the bear, we had the right guys inside making all our Bs, and we really don't need to take anything. We will all need to take some D, because we do not live outside anymore, but we have to adjust that based on where we are on the planet, how much we go outside this year as opposed to last year, how old we are. Every decade we make less D for the same amount of sun exposure. Even if you keep up the same habitual sun exposure every summer, you will inevitably become D deficient in your 60s and 70s.

That means this was always linked to the things that we see in the aging population. It was a normal part of death of all animals. The sleep goes bad. They get constipated. They get a runny nose, and I got rheumatism. My back hurts when I wake up. Those were all things we saw in the elderly. Now they present in young people, but all of these things are correctable. When you use the sleep to correct every single thing that the brain has put off, what I see in my patients makes me think that the brain has a memory of the REM sleep and the slow wave sleep jobs, repair jobs that it put off over the last 20 years.

If you leave a person alone, and you just encourage them to sleep as much as they can, and you get the chemistry right, the body knows what to do, and it will slowly over time correct all the things that have been left off. I do think that are certain people who walk into my office who are in the final stages of cancer, where it's too late, but I don't think that's most of my population. Every single person who's ill in every way, even if you're in the final stages of cancer, you need the best sleep that anybody can give you. That's what you need. You need that and your doctor.

Dr. Gould: There you go. I'm going to want to close the show on that note, how important sleep is. It just makes sense. What did our grandparents tell us? Get a good night's sleep. How do you feel when you've really got a bad night's sleep? You feel terrible. Being used to really crummy sleep isn't the same as having good quality sleep, and I actually know the difference now.

First of all, I would love the right to get you back on the show to talk a little more specifically about some certain things we didn't even get to cover. This is such a fascinating topic, but I want to thank you so much for coming on the show. I'm with you, and I hope we can just wake up the world and say, not all the medicine is wrong, but let's focus on what we can improve without being crazy. Just be reasonable. Thank you so much, and I would love to have you back on the show again.

Dr. Gominak: Thank you, Dr. Gould. I think you're just wonderful, and you're going in the right direction. I'm happy to be a part of that movement. We're making our own movement towards not needing medicines and feeling good, because we sleep well.

Dr. Gould: Fantastic. Thank you so much. You have a great night, and get some good sleep. I know I will as well.

Dr. Gominak: Thank you. Good night.

Dr. Gould: Thank you. Good night. All right, everybody, thank you so much for tuning in. This has been Get Your Smile On with Dr. Joel Gould, your wellness dentist. I'm so excited about all the future things that I'm working on for this podcast, and I can't wait for you all to hear about the incredible things that are really not out there. Until next time, get your smile on, and we'll see you soon. Thank you.

GYSO – Eps. 10
Dr. Krakow PTSD and Insomnia

Dr. Gould: Hello, welcome to Get Your Smile On. I am Dr. Joel Gould, your wellness dentist, broadcasting from beautiful Manhattan Beach, California. Tonight I'm very excited about our show. We have an incredible guest. I want to start at the beginning and just talk about Modern American Dentistry. We have three locations in the Los Angeles area. We like to work with a charity wherever we are, and in our Northridge location we came across a charity called Safe Passage. They are more than just a battered women's shelter. They're actually a program that helps get women back out into the real world and empowers them to reclaim their lives.

I've been working with Trish Steele, and Trish introduced me to Maria DiGiovanni, and this is the producer of our show. She is fantastic. She came to see me, and we did an incredible cosmetic makeover for her, and we used my supermodel crowns. It was a lot of fun. Maris is a very interesting person, and she brought me this show. About the same time I found out that I had sleep apnea, and I started really delving into the world of sleep and trying to get my mind around what was going on with myself and my health.

In one of the podcasts that we did I became interested in Vitamin D as it affects clenching, grinding and sleep. We had Ivor Cummins on our show, and he called in from Ireland. We usually do this show at 7:00PM west coast time, in Ireland we decided that 6:00AM would be a good time to have Ivor on the show, and I said to Maria, "Do you mind doing the show at 10:00PM?" She said, "I don't care. I'm up all night." That really struck a cord with me, because I had been listening to Dr. Steven Park and his podcast, and I had heard an episode of the podcast that had Dr. Barry Krakow on the show, and he is a specialist in PTSD insomnia, and he's a sleep doctor. So we're going to bring him on in just a second, and I'm going to introduce him properly.

Before we do that I just want to go to a quick station break here and thank FoReRadio for having me on this show. Hang on one second, and we'll be right back.

Welcome back. Tonight I'm very excited to have with us Dr. Barry Krakow. He is board certified in internal medicine and board certified in sleep medicine. He also has additional training in emergency and addiction medicine. Dr. Krakow, are you there?

Dr. Krakow: I am here, and I am wide awake. I'm not sleeping.

Dr. Gould: Great. I've got your three books in front of me. You're the author of *Sound Sleep, Sound Mind, Conquering Bad Dreams and Nightmares,* and *Turning Nightmares into Dreams.* I love all those titles. They're really fascinating. First of all, why don't you just tell us a bit about yourself, and what got you interested in sleep.

Dr. Krakow: A number of things got me interested in sleep. One in particular was starting to work with two psychiatrists at the University of New Mexico in 1988. They were doing this fascinating study on nightmare treatment, which everybody would believe is a deeply psychological issue that needs intensive psychotherapy and maybe some heavy duty medication. What we learned was that there are some imagery techniques, just literally what your mind's eye can do in imagination, which can be used to treat chronic nightmares. We published a major article on this showing that even PTSD patients, rape victims, who have awful nightmares, can use this technique and not only improve their nightmares, but it also improves their PTSD. That was published in JAMA in 2001.

My initial entry into sleep medicine was through the field of nightmares. What's so fascinating about that, fast forward, is that we've learned that many nightmare patients have sleep apnea. Obviously nightmare patients would have insomnia too, and we call this the nightmare triad syndrome of nightmares, insomnia, and sleep apnea. Now one of the things that we're researching, this is coming full circle almost 27 years later, we're finding out that if you treat somebody's sleep apnea, whether it's with a dental device, oral appliance therapy, or with positive airway pressure therapy, C-PAP, you'll actually see the nightmares reduce by resolving the breathing disorder.

Dr. Gould: That's pretty fascinating. I know that when I listen to you speak on this subject most people want to think that insomnia is psychological, that they've got some issues, and that they just can't calm down and sleep. What you're basically saying is that there is a real physiological, real medical reason behind a lot of these people's nightmares and their insomnia.

Dr. Krakow: That's correct. It's a very important point that you brought up in terms of the psychological, because that still holds for many patients. In fact, in the most severe patients there tends to be a combination of severe sleep apnea or moderate sleep apnea and severe insomnia. They may benefit from the treatment of the sleep disordered breathing, but then also will need the psychological treatments for insomnia as well. The part that's so fascinating over the last decade is the finding of just how many people only seem to need the PAP therapy or the oral appliance therapy, and then that's it. We even did a study several years ago showing that Breathe Right nasal strips will improve insomnia in people that have mild sleep apnea or what we call upper airway resistance.

So that's pretty amazing that this pathophysiological process is really amenable to different kinds of treatment, and that it seems to affect the psychology as well. The classic example would be if you ask people about what's the single greatest reason they can't sleep at night the answer for 80-90% of them is that they can't turn off their mind. Their mind is racing, racing thoughts, ruminations. Yet at least half of the people with that condition who use PAP therapy as the best example they will actually state that their racing thoughts are gone once they started using PAP therapy. Go figure.

Dr. Gould: I want to sort of slow down here. There's a couple things I want to put out there. A lot of our listeners have come to us through Safe Passage, so we do have a lot of listeners who are PTSD sufferers. My work with Safe Passage has shown me so clearly that even people who've had a lot of abuse and lot of terrible things happen can recover, and that's what Safe Passage is all about. In taking with Maria and some of the other women that I've been dealing with, I'm finding that the majority of these women they all have insomnia, and in fact they all have night terrors too. I kind of wanted you to just help us define what is insomnia or what is chronic insomnia, and then maybe what you've discussed about compound insomnia. Just to give everybody an idea of what we're really talking about. This isn't just sometimes you have a hard time going to sleep.

Dr. Krakow: Right. Some of the basic definitions are that if you have insomnia then you're not sleeping when you want to sleep. It usually takes three forms. You can't fall asleep at night. You wake up in the middle of the night and can't go back to sleep, or you wake up too early, and you can't go back to sleep. Then of course the insomnia has to interfere with your life, in other words, there are people who have broken sleep, but they don't complain about it, for whatever reasons. Maybe they drink 10 cups of coffee a day, and that's why they don't notice the difference. For the people who do notice a difference, the insomnia impacts their life. It impacts the quality of their life. They may have difficulties at work, difficulty in relationships. One of the most obvious things is being tired and irritable from not getting enough sleep and not getting good quality sleep. That's the definition of insomnia, which basically means a broken up periods of sleep, because the person can't either initiate or sustain sleep over what would be thought to be the normal course of the night.

With respect to the sleep terrors, that's actually a very unusual form of parasomnia, and that, of course, in my area of specialty with nightmares is a very interesting area of overlap. Sleep terrors are different than nightmares. Nightmares it's obvious that you had a bad dream. It's obvious that when you wake up you know you had a bad dream, and you almost always know that there's something about the content of the bad dream you remember. So then you can talk to somebody and say, "I had a bad dream. Somebody was chasing me down the alley." A sleep terror is very different, because you could be troubled by disturbing images during the night. You could have your bed partner sleeping next to you and think that you're having this horrible bad dream, but the next morning you wouldn't have any memory of the whole thing, and if the person sleeping next to you tried to wake you up it could actually make things worse, because it's as if you're under threat or under attack when you have a sleep terror. You generally don't try to wake somebody up in that situation.

Dr. Gould: As you're describing this, Maria is messaging me, "Yes, yes, yes." It's incredible, because this is just a recurrent theme for these women, and that's why I was so excited to have you on the show to let them know that there's so much more to this insomnia than just they've had this incredibly horrific experience in their past. I really wanted to bring you on to let them understand that this isn't just all in their heads, and this just isn't something that because they've had these experiences. This is a real and medical issue, and there's really a lot of hope. On this show we've talked a lot about the different topics surrounding sleep disordered breathing. For my regular listeners they know we've sort of been breaking it down, and I'm really looking forward to getting into the more detailed discussion, because this is so far reaching.

I definitely want to speak to you regarding these night terrors. This is something that you saw a lot of. How did that interact with the sleep treatment therapy, the C-PAP therapy, or whatever therapy you're doing to get the airways to be allowing these people to breath? Was there some connection there that was meaningful or useful?

Dr. Krakow: Yeah. In fact it's a great cause for hope based on what you had alluded to earlier, which is that a long time ago, or even as recently as 10 years ago, a lot of people would still think of these PTSD parasomnias, and by the way parasomnia just refers to basically things that go bump in the night, and these parasomnias, whether they're nightmares or sleep walking, sleep terrors, a lot of PTSD patients have these problems, but unfortunately a lot of PTSD patients are not exposed to the evidence in the field of sleep medicine. I had the great fortune to train 20 years ago with Christian Guilleminault at Stanford University who is arguably the world's greatest living sleep researcher. He's published a couple of papers, as have others, showing, remarkably again, that many of these parasomnias are related to breathing disturbances.

I think the easiest way to understand this, even though it hasn't been researched in this fashion, is think about what it would feel like to be choked. It's an awful thing to think about, nobody really wants to spend time imagining it, but think for a moment what is actually the sensation a person would experience if they were choking? In even worse case scenario, think of somebody who was trying to suffocate you and trying to choke you. The answer is that you would feel a tremendous level of threat. I have argued in a couple of places that you can't actually experience a stronger feeling of fear than under the experience of choking. The reason for that is, again not to bring up graphic images, but if somebody was pointing a gun at you you might be extremely scared. There's no question about it, but if somebody was choking you, you would have the belief, the immediate sensation, that you're about to die. That would absolutely have to bring on the greatest possible fear.

What is sleep apnea? Sleep apnea is repetitive choking or mini suffocations all night long. Therefore, as we've said and I've described in my book *Sound Sleep, Sound Mind*, why would somebody who's choking all night long, why would they go to sleep? Why would they ever want to go to sleep knowing about this vulnerability? Of course, the catch is people don't know about this vulnerability, instead their subconscious mind knows about it, and this appears to be the reason, as far as we can tell, again it's not a research point. It's too difficult, but this could be the reason people have racing thoughts. What do racing thoughts do for you at bedtime? They keep you awake. If you are awake, what's not going to happen? You're not going to choke.

This is how this stuff all circles back, and in people who are vulnerable to these parasomnias, like sleep walking, sleep talking, sleep terrors, even nightmares, it may be specifically related to the threat you are experiencing by suffering these mini suffocations. Now treat the mini suffocations, give somebody PAP therapy, oral appliance therapy, the next thing you know the parasomnias are all gone, and that's what Guilleminault described in his papers. The overwhelming number of patients, whether they're with PTSD or not, who report problems like sleep talking, sleep walking, and so on, they declare those symptoms go away once they've been treated for the breathing problem. Breathing's a pretty powerful thing, to say the least.

Dr. Gould:　　I've been talking to a lot of my patients, because I'm seeing this in a lot. We're screening a lot of people here, because I find this so fascinating. To me now the signs are so obvious, but the interesting part of this is when you have these insomnia suffers, and you say, we're going to put a C-PAP on you, what do they say? Is it a complete shock to them, because they're thinking I have a psychological problem, and it's because I've undergone trauma? Are they open to this? Is this a big deal? How does that work?

Dr. Krakow:　　That's a very important question, because at a typical sleep center, where unfortunately the sleep doctors may have little to no training with PTSD, or even little to no training with insomnia or nightmares, there's a sense of throwing up their arms, like what are we going to do with this patient? Certainly they're going to suffer claustrophobia, so why would we expose them to PAP therapy? This is one reason why in the early phases of sleep medicine it became clear that a dental device, oral appliance therapy, could be very useful for some of these people, but then even that proved to be a problem, because some people would then complain, I just can't handle something being inside my mouth.

The bottom line is, if you actually have the time and the patience and the energy and the wherewithal to explain to the PTSD patient that there really is an explanation for why there is so much fragmentation in your sleep, that it isn't just a psychological fragmentation, although that's part of it, but rather there are pathophysiological changes in your breathing that make your brain constantly arousing and awakening all night long. When you show that somebody who is a mental health patient you can actually see them exhibit a sigh of relief, because now they're actually hearing for the first time it isn't really just all in my head. It isn't just psychological. I'm not crazy. There really is a physical explanation for my problem.

Once you can take somebody down that pathway, it's amazing how many PTSD patients become extremely motivated to want to try PAP therapy or dental devices, because they recognize this could make a huge difference in the quality of their sleep. If you try to just give this to somebody, this new movement in sleep medicine called home testing is terrible for mental health patients, because they're going to have the problems that you're alluding to. They're going to take the device. They're going to go home. They're going to try it on. They're going to have a claustrophobic response. They're going to give up, and they're going to say, this is crazy I can't do this. We don't do any of that. We don't do any home testing of PTSD patients.

Dr. Gould: I've got some new data for you. Maria's pretty special. We sent her home with a home sleep tester, just because of the geographic distance that we have, and I know that with Maria she's really open to anything, because we've got a lot of people who are counting on her to be able to bring someone like you on the show and go through this.

Dr. Krakow: Let me just say this. Did she do home testing for the diagnosis or for the treatment?

Dr. Gould: Just for the diagnosis.

Dr. Krakow: Right. There's nothing wrong with that, except that it usually doesn't give as reliable data. I was referring to the people who are sent home with a C-PAP device and a video and the instruction, go use it.

Dr. Gould: What's funny is you're saying that. I've got my regular C-PAP patients here, and there's so many things to discuss about how there's so little care for these people. That's maybe a whole different show, but I can totally see how somebody who has all these issues on top of it all it would be very difficult. It makes perfect sense to see them in more of a clinical setting. This is like a healing for them. I think that sounds completely reasonable to be able to do that.

As Maria was texting me here, we were talking about the avoidance of sleep, and I think that probably a lot of these sufferers hadn't really heard it in these two different ways. Number 1 is, my insomnia is me avoiding feeling like I'm being choked, and Number 2 is, my feeling like I'm being choked or feeling that I'm in danger is real and legitimate. I'm pretty sure we're going to have some pretty reinvigorated people. I actually just wanted to mention this to our listeners that at the end of this show we are going to have the opportunity to take a call or two calls to ask Dr. Krakow any specific questions, and hopefully we'll have some time for that. If that sounds okay with you.

Dr. Krakow: Absolutely.

Dr. Gould: The PTSD part, I guess with the nightmares that basically brought those patients to you then.

Dr. Krakow: Initially the research was all about just the nightmares, and what happened was over the course of that and several other studies on nightmare treatment from 1990 through 1995 we kept repeatedly noticing that nightmare patients were reporting some breathing symptoms. There was snoring, choking, gasping for breath, and we also noticed that at the same time insomnia patients were reporting breathing symptoms.

The part that really sealed the deal for us was that these patients who sometimes didn't report the obvious breathing symptoms would still report what we call end organ symptoms, other kinds of atypical symptoms that nobody would suspect, or clearly suspect, as related to sleep disordered breathing. For example, most people don't realize if you wake up in the morning with a dry mouth it pretty much means you have a sleep breathing disorder, because you're opening your mouth to mouth breath, because you can't get enough air in through your nose. That's a fairly reliable finding. Another one is waking up in the morning with a headache.

The most reliable one, and really an amazing one, is waking up at night to use the bathroom to urinate. The technical term is nocturia. Trips to the bathroom, one of the leading causes of trips to the bathroom, despite what most people think about the prostate or the bladder, are caused directly by sleep apnea. The sleep apnea forces the kidneys to work overtime during the night, and when that happens and you discover that, and you treat somebody, their trips to the bathroom decrease and sometimes go away completely. The person is astonished, and that's a huge motivator, even more motivating than somebody who snores.

A lot of people don't think about snoring, because it's not something they pay attention to, but many people pay attention to waking up at night having to use the bathroom. They're worried about walking in the dark and tripping. They're walking about being awake for too long and having insomnia. It's remarkable how you can use that trips to the bathroom as a very reliable sign of sleep apnea.

Dr. Gould: It's pretty incredible. I know that when people have a hard time believing that they have sleep apnea or that they have what we've talked about, upper airway resistance syndrome, and I see that in a lot of my patients. The thing that convinces them, as it convinced me, myself as a dentist I have a view through a mandibular advancement device. Like most people I'm not thrilled about the idea of wearing a C-PAP, and I'm probably going to at some point use one, but the shock to me was the first night that I wore my MAD I did not get up to go to the bathroom. I always got up to go to the bathroom, and what's funny is as I start to deliver these one by one people who have been having trouble sleeping for a long time they don't wake up the first night and say, "I feel refreshed. I feel great." They all call me and say, "I did not get up to use the bathroom." That's really something else.

I guess it's funny that that would be a great way to make people understand that when they're waking up to go to the bathroom, because my patients all say, "I'm a light sleeper, and I get up to go to the bathroom." I say, "It's your breathing that's probably waking you up, and when you become more conscious you feel the urge to go to the bathroom." As you said, sleep apnea and sleep disordered breathing causes increased urine. I think this is a huge point to make to a lot of our listeners. I'm pretty sure they all have regular bathroom trips. Thank you for bringing that up.

Dr. Krakow: It's a crucial point, Joel, because the exact same thing happened to me in 1998. The very first time I used an oral appliance from Dr. Tom Mead here in Albuquerque, who is a famous inventor of dental devices, the very first night I did not wake up to use the bathroom. I was shocked. What we've learned over the years is that the trips to the bathroom symptom actually seems to reduce before the other daytime symptoms. If you're tired and sleepy, and you're hoping to get benefits from that, you will notice the trips to the bathroom being eliminated before you necessarily feel a lot better during the day. Hopefully that's still enough motivation for the person, but it is fascinating that that particular symptom responds so quickly. Of course, that's great, because it means that the patient is already noticing benefit, and that's going to motivate them.

Dr. Gould: I love it. I think that's great. I want to talk about you and your center in Albuquerque, because I know that you do some special things there. It's not your average sleep center. Why don't you just tell us a little bit about what makes your facility special? For me, what caught my attention is just the attention to the care of your actual technicians who help the patients to work with the actual devices, whether it's an A-PAP or a C-PAP, whatever the latest technology that you guys are using.

Dr. Krakow: Right. We use a lot of advanced technology now called auto bilevel or adaptive servo ventilation. Our center is based on the principle of sleep dynamic therapy, which is the name I've given to the program that we apply at our center. It's described in the *Sound Sleep* book. the idea is to recognize that most sleep disorder isn't just physical or just mental. It's going to almost always be both, and therefore it's very important to lay that out to the foundation right from the beginning so they understand that there is many things that we can do to help. We want to give them as much hope as possible. We want to motivate them as best we can, and we tell them, if you have nightmares we can treat them. If you have insomnia we can treat them. If you have leg jerks and sleep disordered breathing, all of these things can be treated, and they can be treated within just a few months' time, as long we all work together.

With our particular sleep texts at our sleep center, Maimonides Sleep Arts and Sciences, we train them in such a way to give out a lot of this instruction and education to our patients every time they come to the sleep lab. We spend an inordinate amount of time coaching patients to be able to try a cognitive behavioral therapy for insomnia, or learn how to use a different kind of mask to use with PAP therapy. There's just a lot of engagement, and everybody in our center is on board and recognizes that if most of our patients are psychiatric trauma survivors, which is a huge proportion of our population, then we're going to have to be much more attuned to their needs. We do see an occasional classic sleep apnea patient, but that is fairly rare compared to the number of patients who have a psychiatric background.

They're using multiple psychotropic medications. They've been in therapy for 5-25 years. They carry any number of diagnoses, and when they come to us many of them are quite desperate, believing there's nothing that can be done for their sleep. Unfortunately, they were not referred for sleep problems years ago, instead people kept telling them, treat your mental health condition, and your sleep problems will get better. What teach them at our center is, treat your sleep problems, and let's see what it does for your mental health. That's something that they've been thinking about anyway, and that's something they've been expressing to their therapist and their doctors, but a lot of those individuals, unfortunately, are tone deaf and don't understand how important sleep is, but the patients understand how important it is. That's, I believe, one of the main reasons why they end up at our center.

We do get patients from all over the country who come to see us, because they have in fact had these encounters with other mental health professionals, in some cases other sleep doctors, and they're just not making progress.

Dr. Gould: You brought up some amazing points. The one thing I really want to remind my listeners is that the whole idea, the insomnia itself is terrible, but what we're sort of neglecting to mention here is that when you are not getting good and proper sleep, and when you're not getting your REM sleep, your physical body, how you feel emotionally, is suffering, because your body just can't repair itself. These women are dealing with an initial trauma, and now they're dealing with years of poor sleep, and it's not known by the general public and by their doctors that this is actually causing a physical problem. We've talked about this before that it causes anxiety and depression and all manner of hormone mix-ups, because when you can't sleep your body just can't heal. It's incredible what you're doing there.

When we're done with the show, we're going to have one person who wants to come on just to talk to us briefly. I'm going to let Maria announce who she is. I want to let all my listeners know that what I'm trying to do here in Los Angeles is I've been working with Elizabeth Revis, and she deals with victims of violent crime. We really talked about putting together a program here that is going to be accessible for somebody who can't get to Albuquerque for formal help so that there'd be some other options. Dr. Krakow, I wanted to ask you, the Los Angeles area's pretty big, is there anyone here that you work with who you think is doing anything even close to what you're doing? Is there any good referral places out here?

Dr. Krakow: At the risk of sounding very negative, I apologize in advance, but I don't get the impression that there are lot of people who are doing it as comprehensively, in other words, there are sleep centers that clearly know, have cognitive behavioral programs for insomnia and even for nightmares. There are sleep programs that hopefully use the more advanced devices such as the bilevel devices. I know that individually there has to be, for example I know that some people certainly are getting good care at a center like Stanford.

On the other hand, putting it all together the way we've done at our center, I'm actually disappointed and surprised to not hear about more people doing this. It's rather obvious that the comprehensive need of these mental health patients is such that even if you had to have a psychiatrist or psychologist and a sleep specialist all under one roof, so be it. I'm fortunate because I spent almost 15 years training and being mentored by psychiatrists at the University of New Mexico. I've always had an affinity for psychological health. By doing all of my nightmare treatment research I got exposed to having good strong clinical experience with patients. So I'm very comfortable working with virtually all these patients. We even do research, have done research, for the military suicide research consortium on how sleep affects people's suicidal ideation. We're really into it, both because we have a clinical sleep center, and because we have a non-profit research center.

Still I have to say it's been very disappointing to not hear about other programs. The place that it's most burgeoning right now appears to be at specific Army bases around the United States. The last couple of years I've visited Fort Lewis, Fort Bliss, Fort Campbell, Walter Reed, I forget the one in Colorado now, my neighbor. I went to 10 of these bases and gave a three day training program to mental health providers to teach them how to evaluate for both a psychological and the physiological sleep disorders. Many of these bases now are interacting with their own sleep centers.

They're producing their own integrated combination programs, but even there you can sense some of the resistance because it's all about territory. If somebody's doing sleep breathing, well then that must be the pulmonologist. If somebody's doing leg jerks, that must be the neurologist. If somebody's doing insomnia, that must be the psychologist. Unfortunately that's just the way modern medicine has specialized, but that's actually not very good for PTSD patients. They need somebody who does something much more comprehensively and learns how to champion the causes of the PTSD patients.

As you may know from my book and from our research, the average PTSD patient who has a diagnosed case of PTSD is going to have insomnia, is going to have nightmares, is going to have sleep disordered breathing, may also have limb movement disorders such as restless legs, may have circadian rhythm problems, may have anatomical changes in their sinuses and in their nose. It's a pretty broad area of disorders that a PTSD patient's going to suffer from that's clearly not going to be solved by somebody just going into counseling and therapy or just by taking a medication. They need much more, and it is unfortunate that so many either mental health providers on the one hand, or even sleep professionals on the other, are not recognizing these sleep therapy needs in these PTSD patients.

Dr. Gould: I want to stop you there. I want to let you know, first of
               all you have ally in me. I love what you're doing, and
               with me being so involved with Safe Passage I know
               that we're going to be able to put together here in Los
               Angeles to be able to help everybody to get along. What
               I bring to the table, aside from the fact of my own per-
               sonal experience, is that I'm a dentist from Canada. The
               regular rules that apply to a lot of people with their po-
               litical correctness don't apply to me. I'm here to help
               my patients. I'm a holistic dentist with a 'wh', and I look
               at all my patients as a whole.

Dr. Krakow: That's great.

Dr. Gould: Thank you. You've got an ally here, and I've talked with
               some of the women here, and we really want to make
               sure that everybody has a much easier way to get care.
               A lot of what I'm doing in the office is trying to remove
               the access to care, and if that is taking home a take
               home sleep study, if that's what it takes to get some-
               body treated, then that's what we're going to do. I have
               a very clear idea of what I want to do with this whole
               issue, and I really want to raise awareness to the medi-
               cal professionals. That's sort of been my focus. Maybe
               my listeners don't know that I've been working with the
               doctors who don't know what dentists do, don't know
               what sleep doctors do, and don't know what sleep dis-
               ordered breathing is. This is just the tip of the iceberg.

               We're going to be talking about a lot more of this, and
               I just want to mention before we bring Maria on, we've
               got somebody we're going to bring on to talk for one
               second, but Maria is actually in charge of raising aware-
               ness of PTSD in police officers. That's a whole separate
               discussion. We're coming to the end of our time here,
               so I don't want to get slowed down with that, but this
               is so incredible for her to be understanding that some-

body with insomnia and somebody who's dealing with PTSD with police officers, because her abuser was a police officer. So she's doing incredible things for the entire law enforcement community. We're all working together, which is exactly what this issue needs, some working together. Maria, are you there?

Maria:

Yes, I am. Again, both you doctors I want to thank you so much, for me personally and for just to raise awareness to promote this education, because it's such a huge puzzle piece, especially with women who are suffering from PTSD caused by abuse, which I want to bring on a very special guest that's calling in for your show, Dr. Joel. This is Miss Georgia Ambassador for Domestic Sexual Abuse. Marie Waldrop has lost, I'm going to give you away, Marie, I'm so proud. She's lost about 130 pounds, and we're working on about 100 more to go. She keeps going solid, and we thought that may have been why she was suffering from not being able to sleep, but we went a little bit further, and no coincidence want to bring her on, because Dr. Joel, as soon as I met you Marie was going through her own sleep testing at the hospital. I would like to introduce to you right now, Miss Georgia Ambassador for Domestic Sexual Abuse, Marie Waldrop. Marie, here's Dr. Joel.

Marie:

Hi, Dr. Joel.

Dr. Gould:

Hello. We'll say Dr. Barry and Dr. Joel, we'll use our first names. Thank you so much for calling in.

Marie:

You're welcome.

Dr. Gould:

Where are you calling from?

Marie:

I'm calling from Georgia.

Dr. Krakow:

I like that southern accent.

Marie:

Yes. It was kind of funny, because as you were working with Maria about the sleep apnea and stuff I told her, I'm going to the hospital doing the same thing, and they are going to put me on a C-PAP.

Dr. Krakow: That brings up a very important discussion point. I want to make sure you know this fact in case it's relevant to your situation. We have not C-PAP at our center for over a decade. The reason for that is that C-PAP stands for Continuous Pressure. That means you're getting the same pressure whether you breathe in or whether you breathe out. What we've learned is that almost all anxiety patients of any sort need what's called dual pressure, and dual pressure goes by the name of bilevel. What that means is that when you breathe in you get a higher pressure, and when you breathe out you get a lower pressure. So it's much more comfortable. Most people who use C-PAP who feel anxious about it the reason they're feeling anxious about it is because they're trying to breathe out when the air is still coming in. That's why we stopped using C-PAP 10 years ago. One of the things you might want to ask your doctor is whether or not you can try out a bilevel device.

Marie: I'll certainly do that, because I had to talk myself through it, because I don't like anything covering my nose or my mouth, and of course it's tightened around your head and everything. I just had to tell myself it was for my own good and just try to get through it.

Dr. Krakow: Congratulations.

Marie: I was okay until she woke me up that morning and the machine just cut off. When it cut off I kind of freaked out a little bit trying to rip the mask off. I know it had to be a little bit of psychological issue there, but I can't breathe.

Dr. Gould: A little bit? Hold on. A little bit, good for you that you were okay with that. Dr. Krakow's got a very sophisticated program going on, so I think you did great. I'm just so happy that you were open to that. That's a really great sign.

Dr. Krakow: I agree. When are you supposed to get your machine? Do you know?

Marie: I've got to go to Macon next week to see a doctor down there, and he'll talk to me about it. After I see him then I will know about when I'll be able to get it.

Dr. Krakow: Okay. We've already published one study on a very advanced form of this bilevel, and we're actually in the midst of writing up two new research papers on the use of these advanced devices. What I mean by advanced is bilevel itself is advanced, because it gives you two pressures, but these other devices called auto-bilevel or ASV are even more sophisticated, because they are tracking your breathing while you're breathing and adjusting the pressure. So it's called auto-adjusting devices. Again, you may run into sleep doctors who think you don't need it. It's too fancy. It's too expensive, but again we go back to the fact that somebody who is a PTSD patient or somebody who suffers from anxiety we put them in a category of being very sensitive individuals. Therefore what we suspect happens is when they're exposed to the pressure they have very exaggerated responses to it if it has produced some kind of discomfort.

That's a reason we stopped C-PAP, and what we learned is that these other devices, ASV or auto-bilevel is another one, they seem to change the settings every few seconds to accommodate your breathing. We've had much more success. I know we've published an abstract on this just within the last year where we had about 100 PTSD patients using these devices, these auto-bilevel or ASV devices, and roughly 90% of them were able to use the device. Even though many people talk about the

	rate of C-PAP use in PTSD being very low, 90% of this particular sample we looked at was using the device, and we directly think it was related to the sophistication of this technology.
Marie:	They really didn't even give me an option while I was at the hospital. They just said they were going to use that particular machine. I do suffer from anxiety and Post Traumatic Stress Disorder.
Dr. Krakow:	What you can do that is actually reasonable, although it is going to be a little bit difficult for you, is start out with the C-PAP device. Maybe they'll give you some bells and whistles on that device, there's something called auto C-PAP, maybe they'll give you that. That's a little bit better. If you have a good response, that would be great. If the response is not great, then you now have the information to go back and talk to them and say, I tried this device, and I'm struggling with it. These are some of the problems. I actually had a chance to talk to Dr. Krakow about it, and he said that if I had trouble that I should inquire about the possibility, of course be as diplomatic as possible. Doctors don't like to be told what to do by other doctors. Just say, is there any chance I could try one of these newer devices to see if it's more comfortable?
Dr. Gould:	Dr. Krakow, I'm going to break in there and just say, for everyone listening there's a lot of information, and I know that for a lot of the listeners this is the first time they've heard a lot of these details. I want to let everybody know that on our website on Modern American Dentistry when you come onto our site, we will, it's not up yet, we will have an area for you guys to go into specific podcasts where you'll be able to look at the information with Dr. Krakow and any of the other doctors that we've had on, and we're going to have information with the terms and

things that you can talk to your sleep doctors about, because when a doctor has a patient who comes in knowledgeable and empowered I think the results would be great for everybody. We're going to get a better overall picture, not just a doctor saying to a patient, this is what you should do. Just want to close things up a little bit and just let everybody know that we will have that available, and you can come to our website.

Then on that note, first of all I want to say thank you so much for calling in all the way from Georgia. It must be getting late there. We'll say goodbye to you, and then Dr. Krakow I want to close out with you just giving everybody your website, so they can find you right away. As soon as we're offline they can find you right away. Your website's incredible. There's a lot of resources and a lot of great information on this. Why don't you go ahead and tell us how people can get a hold of you?

Dr. Krakow: Our best website is SleepTreatment.com. We have another website, NightmareTreatment.com which is exclusively about nightmare issues, but it will also bring you back to SleepTreatment.com, and you can go in both directions. That has all of the videos. It has information on getting the books, watching certain videos. It tells you how to become a patient if that's something you're interested in. One of the things I'll just close with is that you are correct, Joel, it's not that everybody can make it out to New Mexico, although they probably want to so they can visit Santa Fe, but I'm in Albuquerque, and we do have a Skype program. We call it the Second Opinion Skype Program, and if somebody is having some difficulty and can get referred to us by their local physician, then they can do a Skype appointment with me, and we can try to organize some new strategies for them, regardless of whether they can make it out to New Mexico.

Dr. Gould: Sounds great. That sounds like such a great idea. With computers and technology there's no reason why we shouldn't be doing this, especially since there is such a communication point to this, and not just sending somebody home with a scary machine. Dr. Krakow, I want to thank you so much for coming on this show. I know that we didn't get a chance to talk before, but I knew how important this would be to my listeners, and I know that there's so many people out there who are suffering from this. I'm really sure that people are going to call their friends and say, "Listen to this podcast," because the information that you presented is really groundbreaking.

I know you've been doing this for such a long time that this is normal to you, but to most people, and especially to doctors that are out there, this is completely groundbreaking, and so I want to thank you again, and I want to let you know, as I said, you have an ally in me, and my job is to communicate this message of how all-encompassing sleep disordered breathing is. It's not just sleep apnea. It's so many different things. I want to get you to hang on to the line for one second, and I'm going to say good night to you. Thank you so much. I would love to have you on again in the future.

Dr. Krakow: Thank you so much for having me on the show, Joel.

Dr. Gould: Great. Okay, everybody, thank you for tuning in. I think this was a really incredible and special show. I know it was for me just knowing that I've got Maria who visits my office every two weeks. She makes the trip all the way up from way down south in San Clemente, and we spent a lot of time together, initially thinking that we were going to make over her smile and that was going to be it. There's just so much more, and I just can't tell you how excited I am to have learned this incredible whole different side of PTSD and how it relates to over-all health and to sleeping disorders. Remember that your grandparents probably told you, get a good night's sleep you'll feel much better.

I would like to sign off tonight and say, thank you all for listening. I can't wait to see you all again. I believe we're going to be on break for the next two weeks. I look forward to coming back in September with some new, incredible, and exciting wellness topics. Have a great night.